Notes on Psychiatry

12/75

£ 1.75

I. M. INGRAM M.D., F.R.C. Psych., D.P.M.
Consultant Psychiatrist,
Southern General Hospital, Glasgow
Honorary Clinical Lecturer in Psychological Medicine,
University of Glasgow

G. C. TIMBURY M.B., F.R.C.P.Ed. & Glas., F.R.C. Psych., D.P.M.
Physician Superintendent, Gartnavel Royal Hospital,
Glasgow
Honorary Clinical Lecturer in Psychological Medicine,
University of Glasgow

R. M. MOWBRAY M.A., Ph.D.
Professor of Psychology, Memorial University,
St. John's, Newfoundland

To T. F. R.

Notes on Psychiatry

I. M. INGRAM
G. C. TIMBURY
R. M. MOWBRAY

FOURTH EDITION

CHURCHILL LIVINGSTONE
Edinburgh London and New York 1976

CHURCHILL LIVINGSTONE
Medical Division of Longman Group Limited

Distributed in the United States of America by Longman Inc.,
72 Fifth Avenue, New York, N.Y. 10011, and by associated
companies, branches and representatives throughout the world.

© Longman Group Limited 1976

First edition	1962
Second edition	1964
Third edition	1967
Reprinted	1969
Reprinted	1972
Fourth edition	1976

ISBN 0 443 01334 9

Library of Congress Cataloging in Publication Data

Ingram, Ian Malcolm.
  Notes on psychiatry.

  First-3d editions by T. F. Rodger and others, published under
title: Lecture notes on psychological medicine.
  Includes index.
  1. Psychiatry—Outlines, syllabi, etc. I. Timbury, G. C., joint
author. II. Mowbray, Robert M., joint author. III. Rodger,
Thomas Ferguson. Lecture notes on psychological medicine.
IV. Title [DNLM: 1. Mental disorders. WM100 153n]
RC457.153 1975   616.8′9   75-17741

Printed in Great Britain

Preface

These notes are deliberately concise. They are suitable for revision, but as an introduction must be supplemented by lectures, clinical experience and further reading (see p. 125). They first appeared in 1962 and were compiled for medical students at the University of Glasgow. Over the years they have been found useful, not only by medical undergraduates, but by medical postgraduates requiring to revise psychiatry quickly for the M.R.C.P., or when first entering psychiatric practice, and by students of nursing, health visiting, social work, psychology and occupational therapy.

Despite many revised reprints and several new editions it has been found necessary to recast and rewrite most of the text. Several new chapters have been added.

Glasgow,   I.M.I.
1975

Contents

1. Psychopathology

In psychiatry the patient's mental state is described in a mixture of everyday and technical terms. Sometimes everyday words are used in a special or more precise sense, e.g. 'delusion', 'confusion'. The study and description of the patient's subjective experience is called psychopathology or phenomenology. It is invaluable in *understanding* the patient's experience but is not objective and does not *explain* the symptoms. To find causes we must look for explanations in genetic, metabolic and environmental factors.

Common abnormalities

1. *Disorders of perception*

    a. *Illusions.* Objects perceived are distorted and falsely interpreted, e.g. pictures in the fire, trees in the dark taking on human shape.

    b. *Hallucinations* are perceptions arising without external stimulus. They may be auditory (hearing voices when no one is speaking), visual (visions), or somatic, e.g. bodily sensations of sexual interference. They should be distinguished from pseudo-hallucinations which usually occur in hysteria and lack conviction, e.g. the patient sees things in his 'mind's eye' or with his eyes closed. *Hypnagogic or hypnopompic hallucinations* (while falling asleep or waking) are not necessarily pathological.

    c. *Déjà vu* is one of various abnormalities of imagery. The person has a strong sense of familiarity on encountering a strange place or person. Occurs in some normals and in temporal lobe epilepsy.

2. *Disorders of thinking*

    It is crucial to distinguish *form* and *content* of thought, i.e. what is thought (the content) and the way in which it is thought (the form). *Formal thought disorder* refers to disorder of form.

a. *Concrete thinking:* inability to think conceptually or abstractly. Tested by interpretation of proverbs. A person with concrete thinking cannot give the general meaning of a proverb, e.g. 'A drowning man will clutch at a straw' — 'He could breathe through it'; an ingenious but concrete response.

b. *Dereistic thinking:* thinking determined by mood and instinct which disregards reality, e.g. wish-fulfilling day dreams.

c. *Acceleration* (pressure of thought, flight of ideas) and *retardation.*

d. *Perseveration:* the persistence of thoughts and actions after they have served their purpose, e.g. patient may respond to a new question or instruction by repeating his response to the previous one.

e. *Circumstantiality:* overdetailed and roundabout thinking; inability to separate the important from the trivial.

f. *Incoherence:* thinking and speech may show *fragmentation* or *contamination* (words or parts of words fused).

3. *Delusions*

A delusion is a belief which cannot be accepted by others of the same class, education or cultural background and which cannot be changed by logical argument or evidence against it. The hallmarks of a true delusion are the overwhelming conviction with which it is held and its incorrigibility, even when it is absurd.

a. *Secondary delusions* are psychologically understandable as arising from (secondary to) some other abnormality such as thought disorder or mood disturbance; e.g. a depressed patient may believe that he has committed an unforgivable sin, despite a relatively blameless life. The delusion is secondary to the disturbed mood.

b. *Primary delusions* are psychologically incomprehensible and not derived from other psychological states. They are often preceded by a feeling of 'delusional atmosphere' or 'awareness' — a feeling of impending revelation.

c. *Delusional perceptions and misinterpretations.* Things are seen or heard normally, but special significance is attached to them. *Delusional memories* also occur.

d. *Overvalued ideas:* may be confused with delusions. They are convictions which can be understood in the light of the person's background and personality: usually propagated or defended in a fanatical way.

4. *Disorders of emotion (affect)*

a. *Depression* and *elation* may be understandable or non-understandable. The central disturbance is of vitality (increased or diminished) and is often experienced both physically and mentally.

b. *Apathy:* loss or absence of feeling.

c. *Depersonalisation:* the feeling that one has lost one's feelings; a feeling of not being real.

d. *Derealisation:* the feeling that objects and people no longer seem real, that no feeling is experienced towards them.

e. *Anxiety* and *ecstasy* are other variations in mood.

5. *Compulsive phenomena*

a. *Obsessions:* contents of consciousness from which the person cannot free himself, although he recognises them to be nonsensical or groundless. He feels compelled to think them and at the same time tries to resist them.

b. *Compulsions:* acts which the person feels compelled to carry out, e.g. touching, washing, against his own resistance and with knowledge that they are senseless.

6. *Disorders of consciousness*

Between the normal states of sleep/waking and the severe abnormality of coma there are various disorders of consciousness. In most there is *clouding of consciousness* characterised by disturbed awareness of time, place and person (disorientation). *Torpor* is a state of pathological drowsiness with clouding of consciousness. *Delirium* is the term used when physical restlessness is added. In *twilight states* the patient may appear to behave normally, but has only cloudy recall on recovery. Attention is usually narrowed and situations incompletely understood.

7. *Disorders of memory*

Four elements of memory can be disordered: grasp, retention, recall, and recognition. Immediate and long-term memory may be separately disturbed. *Amnesia* can occur in delirious states or in clear consciousness. If grasp and retention are intact and recall alone impaired an emotional cause is likely (hysterical amnesia). Head injury may produce *retrograde* amnesia. *Confabulation:* in amnesic states the patient may confabulate, i.e. invent material to fill gaps in his memory.

2. Classification of Psychiatric Disorders

Normal/abnormal?

In medicine we tend to interpret normal and abnormal as synonyms for healthy and sick and to consider the difference as quite distinct, as an all or none phenomenon rather than as a continuum.

In normal and abnormal behaviour — the subject matter of psychology and psychiatry — other usages are found. Not only can normal and abnormal mean healthy and sick, they can mean responsible and irresponsible (a legal interpretation), good and bad (a moral interpretation), or average and deviant (a statistical interpretation based on the normal distribution curve).

Psychiatric signs and symptoms are best regarded as deviations from average behaviour and experience. This statistical usage is neutral and does not imply sickness, irresponsibility, or immorality. The idiot and the genius are both extreme deviations from an average, and are therefore both *statistically abnormal,* but in terms of pathology only the idiot would be recognised as sick.

Normal and abnormal behaviour must also be placed in their social, cultural and historical context. What was normal behaviour 100 years ago may seem strange today: what is acceptable in one social class may seem strange in another, and what is tolerated in one community or country may lead to hospital admission or arrest elsewhere.

Because the standards for normality are complex, and the abnormal is not necessarily pathological, the division between health and disease is less clear-cut in psychiatry than in other branches of medicine. It is mainly in psychiatry that patients are found who do not accept that they are unwell, or who regard themselves as sick or wicked when the doctor does not.

Classification

In general medicine most illnesses can be classified on the basis of their aetiology, pathology, or relationship to a system of the body. In some psychiatric disorders, e.g. those due to cerebral syphilis and atherosclerosis, the same applies, but in the bulk of psychiatric disorders the causes are multiple, a combination of genetic, social and environmental factors, or not precisely known. As a result most psychiatric classification is descriptive and based on observation of symptoms, signs and the natural history of the disorder. Such a classification is crude and not entirely reliable: psychiatrists have been shown to agree reliably on the broad categories of diagnosis but to be less consistent in the specific labels they attach to patients.

Three broad lines of demarcation are used:

1. The main division of mental disorders is into *mental illness* and *mental handicap* (deficiency, subnormality). Mental handicap is a condition which includes intellectual deficit and has been present from birth or an early age. Mental illness implies previous health: a disorder developing or manifesting itself later in life. The division is a very old one and has been perpetuated by legislation and by the use of separate hospitals for mental illness and mental handicap. In English law psychopathy (see p. 52) is regarded as a separate category.

2. The principal division of mental illness is into *psychoneurosis* and *psychosis.* These categories correspond to lay notions of 'nerves' and 'madness'. The psychoneuroses are common conditions whose symptoms seem understandable and can be empathised with. The psychoses are illnesses in which the symptoms are less understandable, cannot be empathised with, and in which the patient often loses contact with reality. The distinction is crude, and has exceptions, but is serviceable.

3. The terms *functional* and *organic* refer to the aetiology of the disease and are used to sub-divide the psychoses. Functional psychoses are those in which function is disturbed but no pathology can be demonstrated with current methods. Diagnosis of an illness as functional should rest on finding positive psychological symptoms and not merely upon exclusion of physical findings. Organic psychoses are those in which a demonstrable or inferred lesion is present, e.g.

tumours, vascular changes, infective, toxic, traumatic or congenital factors.

Nomenclature

Variations exist, and are given in brackets, all being in common use.

Psychoneuroses
Anxiety neurosis, phobic states, hysteria, obsessional neurosis, post-traumatic neurosis.

Functional psychoses
Affective: manic-depressive psychosis (depression or mania).

Schizophrenia: paranoid, hebephrenic, catatonic, simple.

Organic psychoses (symptomatic psychoses)
Acute (delirium), subacute (dysmnesic syndrome, subacute delirious state), chronic (dementia), atypical.

Personality disorders

Psychosomatic disorders

Mental handicap (subnormality)
Organic, subcultural.

FURTHER READING

A Glossary of Mental Disorders: Studies on Medical and Population Subjects,
    No. 22. (1968) London: H.M.S.O.

3. The Psychiatric Interview

The student may experience difficulties in his first encounters with psychiatric patients. Some of these difficulties arise from the nature of psychiatric symptoms and signs: disorders of emotion, of thinking, or of intelligence are less easy to elicit and describe than physical signs and symptoms. The interviewer may have to overcome his own anxieties and preconceptions about the mentally ill. Lastly, the range of information which is sought about the patient and his illness is much wider than for other clinical disciplines and requires tact, time and patience to elicit.

Nevertheless, the clinical approach is fundamentally the same as in other subjects. A methodical approach leading to a formulation of the case, which details diagnosis, prognosis and treatment, is the ultimate goal of all investigation of the patient.

During his instruction each student should interview patients and their relatives if possible, record his findings and discuss them with his teachers. In no area of medicine is practical experience more necessary, and theory less helpful.

Interviewing

The psychiatric interview is used both for investigation and psychotherapy (see p. 103). For the patient, giving a detailed and frank account of his life and problems may in itself have a therapeutic effect. The interviewer must form a good relationship with the patient and at the same time study the patient and the relationship. He is a participating observer and needs to be constantly alert to what the patient is saying and how he is behaving. The techniques necessary vary with the doctor's own personality and can be learned only by constant practice with a wide range of patients combined with self scrutiny.

The student should aim to discover the pattern of the illness, the exact nature and origin of the symptoms and to place these in the setting of the patient's personality and life history. The case history is both descriptive and developmental. The interview should cover all the material in the scheme of case taking and this may require a series of interviews. The order given need not be followed rigidly in the interview but should be adhered to in recording it. It is sensible to start the interview with the patient's present complaints rather than a detailed enquiry about his or her family history. Interviewing can be directive or non-directive and the initial investigating interview should strike a balance between direct questioning and allowing the patient to tell his story in his own way. Leading questions and interruptions should be avoided but the interview should be guided by asking for particular instances rather than generalisations and by changing the trend with comments and questions.

Recording

Make full notes at the time using the patient's own words and expressions where possible. As soon as possible after the interview the notes should be expanded and written up in terms of the scheme shown. The final case record should be legible and clearly set out. It is vital to record negative information as well as positive items. The mental state should give a vivid account of the patient's behaviour at the time of the interview and a provisional formulation and diagnosis must be made. This may require revision later but is a useful discipline. In all cases it is helpful to obtain further history from a relative. All notes should be signed.

Scheme of case-taking

Several interviews with a patient are usually required to complete this scheme. Where only one interview is undertaken it will be necessary to abbreviate the scheme.

Case-taking is divided into:

1. History of present illness
2. Social and personal history (supplementary history to be obtained from relative if possible)

3. Physical examination
4. Psychiatric examination (mental state)
5. Further investigations
6. Formulation.

1. History of present illness

State briefly mode of referral/admission, reason for admission and patient's complaints (in his own words), and their duration. Patient's attitude to the illness and to the referral should also be noted. Also state if a relative or friend has been seen.

Give a detailed, coherent account, in chronological order, of the illness from the earliest time at which a change was noticed until the present. Give data which will permit the onset and sequence of various symptoms to be dated as accurately as possible.

2. Social history

Family history
  Father: health, age, or age at time of death, and cause of death. Personality. Occupation.
  Mother: health, age, or age at time of death, and cause of death. Personality. Occupation.
  Siblings: enumerate in chronological order of birth with Christian names, ages, marital status, personality, occupation, state of health (miscarriages and stillbirths to be included).
  Social position and general efficiency of family. Any familial diseases, alcoholism, abnormality of personality, mental disorder, epilepsy. (If unknown or none say so.) Extend this investigation beyond the immediate family, e.g. to grandparents, uncles, aunts, cousins. Note particulars which might be required for further enquiries, e.g. names of hospitals where relatives have been treated.
  Home atmosphere and influence: any important events for parents or other members of the household. Emotional relationship to parents, siblings, and relatives.

Personal history
  Date and place of birth: mother's condition during

pregnancy. Any complications of pregnancy or delivery. Birth weight. Breast or bottle fed.

Early development: delicate or healthy baby. Precocious or retarded. Time of teething, talking, walking, toilet training.

Neurotic symptoms in childhood: night-terrors, sleep-walking, tantrums, bed-wetting, thumb-sucking, nail-biting, faddiness about food, stammering, mannerisms, anxieties (specify).

Health during childhood: infectious diseases, chorea, infantile convulsions, etc.

School: age of beginning and finishing. Standard reached. Evidence of ability or backwardness. Special abilities or disabilities. Hobbies and interests. Relationship to school-mates and teachers. Games.

Adolescence: attitudes to family and authority. Re-belliousness. Friendships or solitary. Fantasy life.

Occupations: age of starting work. Jobs held in chronological order, with ages, dates, reasons for change. Present economic circumstances. Ambitions. Satisfaction in work or reasons for dissatisfaction. Military service: experience, promotion, reaction to stress.

Sexual history: age at onset of puberty (menarche, shaving); reactions. Masturbation. Fantasies. Experience. Disorders and deviations. Current outlets. Contraception.

Marriage: date of marriage, age, health and personality of spouse. Length of courtship. Marital relations.

Children: chronological list of children, giving ages, names, personality and health. Attitudes to children. Have there been miscarriages?

Habits: food, sleep, alcohol, tobacco, drugs (especially analgesics, hypnotics). Specify any change in habits.

Medical history: illnesses, operations, accidents and hospital attendances, chronologically and with details.

Previous mental illness: dates, duration, symptoms of attacks: in what hospital or out-patient department. Treatment received and response to treatment. Names and addresses of hospitals and doctors.

Antisocial behaviour: any history of violence, gambling, delinquency or criminal behaviour. Convictions, periods in Borstal or prison.

Current life situation: summary of patient's domestic and work circumstances at present time. Recent stresses or emotional conflicts of any kind.

Personality before illness

Social relations: to family, to friends and workmates. Was he/she leader, follower or organiser, aggressive, submissive, adjustable, dependent, etc?

Activities and interests: groups, societies, clubs, hobbies, books, radio, T.V., cinema.

Mood: describe in terms such as cheerful, despondent, anxious, worrying. Was he/she self-deprecating, satisfied, over-confident, stable, fluctuating (with or without any reason), controlled, demonstrative.

Character: describe in terms such as timid, sensitive, suspicious, resentful, quarrelsome, irritable, impulsive, jealous, selfish, egocentric, reserved, shy, self-conscious, strict, fussy, rigid. Give examples.

Standards: moral, religious, social, economic, practical. Attitude towards self, others, health and bodily functions.

Energy and initiative: output sustained or fitful. Easily fatigued, daily rhythm, sleep habits, ability to make decisions.

Reaction to stress: level of tolerance, types of stress (frustration, loss) and response (anger, depression). Typical or excessive defence mechanisms. Personality defects revealed by stress.

3. Physical examination

Physical examination should be comprehensive and should be carried out within a day of admission. Special attention should be given to the central nervous system. Positive and negative findings should be recorded and a brief summary of abnormalities found should be given. When possible physical examination should precede assessment of the mental state, as observation of the patient's behaviour during this examination is often informative or revealing.

4. Psychiatric examination (mental state)

General behaviour: appearance, ward behaviour since

admission, and attitude to hospital, nurses, doctors, other patients. Activity. Eating and sleeping.

Talk: (describe its form here, not its content.) Much or little. Spontaneous or only in answer to questions. Rate, coherence. If abnormal, give *sample of talk*.

Mood: not only happiness or sadness but irritability, perplexity, fear or anxiety. Constancy and causes of variations. Appropriate or incongruous. Attitude to future. Suicidal thoughts.

Form of thought: ability to think in abstract terms (test with proverbs and record answers) consistently and without interruption of flow. Does patient experience blocking, pressure or poverty in thinking?

Content of thought: describe in detail the content of thought, problems and preoccupations. List main worries.

Delusions and misinterpretations. Doubts about environment. Ideas of reference, persecution. Are there delusions of self-depreciation, grandiosity, guilt, hypochondriasis, poverty, etc.

Hallucinations and other disorders of perception (auditory, visual, tactile, etc.). Manner of reception, source, vividness, occurrence. Alone? At night? Feelings of unreality or changes in the self (derealisation or depersonalisation).

Obsessional phenomena: content of obsessions and extent to which they are resisted. Recognition of their absurdity. Relation to emotional state. Association with compulsive acts and rituals.

Orientation: knowledge of name, identity, place, time, date, other persons and circumstances of admission.

Memory: estimate from patient's account of history. Test for recent and remote events, recall of a list of numbers and of a name and address — immediately and after five minutes. Immediate recall of sentence, e.g. 'The one thing a nation needs in order to be rich and great is a large secure supply of wood.' Note repetitions required to learn the sentence.

Attention and concentration: easily distracted? Preoccupied? Tests: Days and months in reverse order. Serial 7's. (Subtract 7 from 100, then from 93 and so on until 2 is reached.)

General information: test according to patient's experience and education and estimate with these in mind, e.g. using current events, Prime Minister, Royal Family, capital cities and large towns, etc.

Intelligence: estimate from history and general knowledge. Note discrepancies between this estimate and the patient's educational and occupational background.

Insight and judgement: attitude to present state. Regarded as illness? In need of treatment? Plans for future. Attitude to ... ...mestic or ethical problems present.

.. Note staff reactions to patient's behaviour. interview, interviewer's reactions.

...tigations

...igations as indicated.

...testing.

...:ial worker's report.

...of the case

...fferential diagnosis, giving evidence for and ...ous possibilities. Make and record a *pro-*
...s, an estimate of prognosis, a *problem list,*
...her investigation and *treatment.*

4. Psychological Tests

Various tests are used in the examination of the psychiatric patient in order to measure aspects of intelligence or of personality. The administration and scoring of these tests requires expertise and in practice patients are referred to specially trained clinical psychologists who undertake testing as one part of their hospital duties. Clinical psychologists also undertake Behaviour Therapy with certain patients (see Chap. 21).

Intelligence tests

Tests of general intelligence yielding an intelligence quotient (IQ) are used:

1. In the diagnosis of mental handicap
2. To provide background information about the patient for diagnosis and prognosis
3. In the assessment of the patient for rehabilitation and vocational guidance.

For example, an IQ may help to decide whether a patient's difficulty at work is due to a discrepancy between his intelligence and what is expected of him, or is due to emotional difficulties. The patient's test results are appraised in the light of his educational, occupational and social history.

Examples

Wechsler Adult Intelligence Scale. The IQ is derived from the results of 11 sub-tests. Six of these tests are verbal (i.e. question and answer) and five are performance tests (involving manipulation of test material).

Verbal tests

Vocabulary (defining words)
Information (general knowledge)
Comprehension (commonsense)

Arithmetic (14 mental calculations)

Similarities (categorising similarities between pairs of items)

Digit span (remembering increasing sequences of numbers).

Performance tests

Digit symbol (substituting symbols for numbers)

Picture completion (noting missing items in drawings)

Block design (reproducing diagrams using coloured blocks)

Picture arrangement (arranging pictures in logical sequence)

Object assembly (jigsaws).

This scale yields:

1. An overall measure of intellectual capacity

2. Separate measures of intelligence on verbal and performance scales

3. Indication of the patient's particular intellectual abilities or defects

4. An estimate of the degree of intellectual deterioration.

Progressive Matrices. This test measures intellectual ability using the capacity to reason by understanding relationships. The patient is asked to select from a number of alternatives the design which completes a pattern. Sixty such problems of increasing difficulty are presented to the patient. His score on the test when corrected for age yields a percentile rating (i.e. his relative position for intelligence in a random sample of 100 members of the population).

The test is useful as a quick indicator of a patient's level of intelligence. Because it is non-verbal and self-explanatory it can be used in patients with speech or language difficulties.

The Progressive Matrices gives a measure of general intelligence only when it is combined with a score on the Mill-Hill Vocabulary Scale (a standard list of words arranged in order of difficulty, each of which has to be defined).

Measuring intellectual deterioration

In psychiatric illnesses various types of intellectual handicap may occur (see Chap. 6). In dementia the intellectual loss may be assessed clinically by comparing the patient's present performance with the pre-illness level of functioning judged from school and occupational history. A more accurate measurement of intellectual deterioration can be achieved by using the results of the tests which are known to be resistant to intellectual loss, for example vocabulary tests as indicators of the pre-illness level of intelligence, and noting the discrepancy between these resistant test-scores and the scores on tests which are sensitive to deterioration. For example, comparing the patient's score on Mill-Hill Vocabulary Scale (resistant) with his score on Progressive Matrices (sensitive) gives a measure of the degree of intellectual deterioration over and above that expected for his age.

In addition, special tests are used to elicit specific intellectual changes such as: memory loss (Wechsler Clinical Memory Scale and Benton Visual Retention test), perceptual disturbances (Bender Gestalt test), disturbance of abstract thinking (Goldstein Scherer test).

The *Halstead-Reitan Neuropsychological Test Battery* consists of a large number of tests of the patient's intellectual, motor and speech functions. It includes tests of thinking, orientation, perception of rhythm and speech, tactile recognition, aphasia as well as general intelligence and takes several hours to administer to a patient. Performance on all the individual tests is combined to give an index of intellectual impairment and analysis of results can give indications of localisation of the central nervous system lesion.

The *Crichton Geriatric Scale* consists of a group of tests designed to discriminate between functional and organic conditions in the elderly. As well as containing a standard IQ test for the elderly, this scale includes an orientation test and a test measuring the patient's ability to detect simultaneous two-point sensory stimulation (the Face-Hand test).

Tests of thinking

Two tests in common use which are designed to measure abnormal thinking in schizophrenic patients are the *Payne Classification Test* and the *Bannister Grid Test for Schizophrenic Thought Disorder*. The former is made up of a number of objects, varying according to size, shape, colour, etc., which the patient is asked to group in any way he likes. There are a number of acceptable (normal) groupings, and any grouping outwith this is termed 'overinclusive', and indicates that the person is using a wide and unusual classificatory system when he thinks.

The *Bannister Repertory Grid Test* measures how well integrated and consistent a person's thinking is. It consists of a number of pictures of male and female faces which the patient is required to order according to the degree to which they possess certain personality traits, e.g. kind, sincere, etc. This test correlates highly with psychiatric ratings of thought disorder in schizophrenic patients, who typically show loose and inconsistent thinking on this test.

Personality tests

Questionnaires

The patient can be asked to complete or tick answers to a list of questions about his attitudes, habits and ways of behaving. For example, the *Eysenck Personality Inventory* (E.P.I.) presents 57 questions to be ticked 'Yes' or 'No' and the answers are analysed in terms of the personality characteristics, neuroticism and extraversion. Recently Eysenck has added a new scale to this which he calls psychotism. Questionnaires are generally too inaccurate for individual clinical work but may be of value in investigating the personality characteristics of groups of patients. Many others are in use, some measuring diagnostic categories and others personality traits.

The *Minnesota Multiphasic Personality Inventory* (M.M.P.I.) is used in psychiatric diagnosis. The patient is asked to judge whether each of 550 statements applies to himself. These statements cover a wide spectrum of mental and somatic complaints, habits, attitudes and moods. The patient's responses are converted into a profile covering 10 basic scales such as Depression, Paranoia, Hysteria, etc. A scoring method is available to detect exaggeration or bias in the responses given by the patient.

The *Sixteen Personality Factor Test* (16 P.F.) measures 16 common personality traits. Unlike the M.M.P.I. scales these are not psychiatric but are psychological characteristics, such as self-sufficiency, submissiveness, imaginativeness, radical-mindedness, etc. These traits are derived statistically from a factor analysis of 185 questions answered on a Yes/No/Uncertain basis. For each individual an overall personality profile is obtained.

While the 16 P.F. assesses surface traits, the *Edwards Personal Preference Schedule* (E.P.P.S.) attempts to assess an individual's psychological needs. This test measures such characteristics as a need for achievement, need for autonomy, need for order, etc. This need profile may be compared with the actual surface trait profile obtained from the 16 P.F.

Other questionnaires try to assess a single personality trait with a high degree of accuracy. Examples of these are the *Fould's Hostility* and *Hysteroid Scales*.

Projective tests

The patient is presented with unstructured or meaningless material such as inkblots (Rorschach test) or vague pictures (Thematic Apperception test) and asked to report what he perceives. The patient's responses to this material are considered to be projections of himself from which the examiner can make inferences about personality. While interesting responses may be obtained, their interpretation is difficult and unreliable, and these tests are less widely used than formerly.

FURTHER READING

Cattell, R. B. *Scientific Analysis of Personality*. Penguin.
Gathercole, C. E. *Assessment in Clinical Psychology*. Penguin.
Mowbray, R. M. & Rodger, T. F. *Psychology in Relation to Medicine*. Churchill Livingstone.
Williams, M. *Brain Damage and the Mind*. Penguin.

5. Epidemiology

The study of disorders in groups and communities is of obvious importance in psychiatry: first, because multiple causes may more readily be investigated in this way; second, because environmental factors are relevant to many psychiatric conditions; and third, because positive findings may lead to social preventive measures.

Prevalence of psychiatric disorder

For over a century contemporary stresses ranging from railway travel to atomic warfare have been blamed for apparent increases in mental illness. These increases have, however, been in hospital admission rates and research indicates that increased admissions follow increased provision of hospital beds; changes in legislation have made treatment more easily available and have diminished the stigma attached to it. In the last 40 years the development of effective physical treatments has encouraged admissions.

There is little evidence that the true prevalence of psychiatric disorders has changed greatly in the last century, except for the increases in affective illness and dementia associated with the general aging of the population.

Prevalence today can be measured by admission rates, by outpatient attendances, by psychiatric patients seen in general practice and by community surveys. One careful study in general practice showed that of all patients seen, 15 per cent had mild, 3 per cent moderate, and 1.4 per cent severe psychiatric disorders. A further 13 per cent were considered to show some emotional disturbance, making a total of one-third of all patients. A hospital census in England showed that on one day 2.86 per 1000 of the population were hospitalised for psychiatric reasons. Of these, 31 per cent were mentally handicapped and 69 per cent mentally ill. It has been estimated that the individual's lifetime expectancy of a psychiatric admission is 5 per cent.

Other epidemiological findings

Specific findings about suicide, schizophrenia and affective illness will be found in the appropriate chapters but the following findings have some general importance:

Sex. Females have higher admission rates than males.

Age. Admission rates increase with age up to the seventies.

Marital status. Marriage protects against admission, shortens stay, and increases the chances of discharge.

Urban/rural. Rates are higher in town than in country. The larger the city, the higher the rates.

Migration. Immigrants and emigrants have higher rates.

National and cultural. Primitive communities are not immune although the culture may colour the symptomatology. There are no major variations among western countries.

Social class. Has been studied in detail for many conditions. Mental illness has a social geography. In the decaying centres of the big cities schizophrenia is more prevalent, and this and other disorders (but not affective illness) are associated with areas of social disorganisation and mobility. Schizophrenia is six times as common in social class five as in social class one, but the increase is due to 'drift' of patients down the social scale — a consequence of illness rather than its cause.

Conclusions

Epidemiological studies of psychiatric disorder and of suicide demonstrate that social disorganisation and isolation are associated with high risks of breakdown. Those at risk in the community include the elderly, those widowed and divorced, the unmarried, and those living alone or away from home, especially in large cities.

FURTHER READING

Arthur, R. J. *An Introduction to Social Psychiatry.* Penguin.
Kiev, A. *Transcultural Psychiatry.* Penguin.

6. Organic States and Epilepsy

Definition of organic states

Organic mental illnesses are caused by anatomical or physiological disturbance occurring primarily in the brain or central nervous system or resulting from physical illness elsewhere in the body. Acute organic states are sometimes called symptomatic psychoses; chronic states are referred to as dementias. The symptomatology varies with the rate of development of the disease process, the position, duration, extent and severity of the damage to the central nervous system, and the premorbid personality and intelligence of the patient.

'Organic' pathology should be suspected where psychiatric symptoms occur in the presence of the following:

1. No positive emotional factors in aetiology
2. History of trauma, toxic factors, familial degenerative disease, etc.
3. Abnormal neurological signs
4. Age over 45 years.

Certain psychological changes are characteristic, e.g. sudden or progressive deterioration of intellectual powers, especially memory, beyond that expected for age and basic intelligence; loss of sensory or motor function; perceptual changes, e.g. loss of spatial perception; disorientation; sudden or progressive change of personality, especially the following — inappropriate mood, euphoria, apathy, lack of concern for others, shallowness of affect, bizarre behaviour, misinterpretations, 'moral deterioration', irritability, 'catastrophic reactions', 'organic orderliness'.

Examination and investigations

A full history should be obtained from the patient and a friend or relative.

Both psychiatric and neurological examinations should be undertaken. Special attention should be paid to the following features:

Appearance and general behaviour. Consistent with history? Mannerisms, tics, posture. Tidiness and appropriateness of dress.

Mood. Appropriate to the situation. Emotional lability or fixity. Insight. Disinhibition.

Orientation. Time, date, place, person, age, circumstances of hospitalisation. Can he estimate time-intervals and experience continuity in time? Can he orientate himself readily in new surroundings?

Attention. Distractibility or imperturbability. Can he shift from one topic to another? Is his concentration impaired? Does he perseverate?

Memory. Does memory seem intact? Can he remember events of an hour ago, a day ago? Can he remember more remote events? Nature of amnesia, e.g. for names, faces, and whether it is retrograde or anterograde. Confabulations and fabrications. Does spontaneous recall differ from deliberate recall?

Intelligence. General impression. Range of knowledge and expression. Test reading, writing, comprehension. Are abilities consistent with education and level of intelligence? Agraphia, alexia, acalculia. Can he use numbers as concepts?

Speech. Clarity, modulation, articulation, pronunciation, stammering, aphasia, dysphasia range of vocabulary and use of words.

Thinking. Abstract and concrete thinking. Can he control the direction of his thinking? Note content.

Personality. In what way has the personality changed from premorbid personality? Interests, motives, inter-personal relationships, ethical sense.

Tests of intellectual deterioration (see p. 18).

Detailed physical examination of the nervous system with Wasserman test, lumbar puncture, skull X-ray, EEG, perimetry, angiography, EMI scan, etc., as indicated.

Clinical descriptions

In the symptomatic psychoses the most important symptom

is *clouding of consciousness*. This is a state of disturbed awareness which may vary from coma to the mildest degree of confusion. EEG changes are present in proportion to the degree of clouding.

Acute organic states

Delirium. Symptomatic psychoses in which consciousness is clouded to the extent that the patient is disorientated for time and place. The attention is fleeting and narrowed — the patient is unable to grasp his present situation and relate it to the past. Thinking is concerned with imaginary experiences and there may be illusional falsifications and dream-like hallucinations — usually visual. Restlessness and hyperkinesis occur; in extreme cases, muttering delirium. Speech disturbance such as pointless repetition, perseveration and dysarthria are found. The mood is one of fear and bewilderment. Sleep rhythm is disturbed. There may be fits.

In each case the individual pattern, especially the thought content, is determined by the premorbid personality. After recovery there is usually amnesia for the events of the illness. Residual delusions may occur and a paranoid attitude may persist for some time.

Subacute organic states

Dysmnesic syndrome. The principal symptom is a difficulty in retaining recent events. There is vague and faulty orientation, and a varying degree of confabulation. Delirium may return at night. This picture may last from a few days to several months, and often follows a delirium.

Subacute delirious state. A symptomatic psychosis in which the degree of clouding is less deep and less constant than in delirium. Incoherence of thought and speech appear, together with perplexity, in a setting of clouding of consciousness which fluctuates in degree and is worse at night. The illness may last for weeks but normally ends in recovery.

Chronic organic states

Dementia. Usually defined as an irreversible decline of mental functions produced by organic brain disease. The process may be arrested; e.g. in neurosyphilis, vitamin deficiencies, some brain tumours. The most obvious finding is intellectual deterioration, but emotion and volition are also impaired. The earliest changes are difficulty in recent memory, failing attention and slow, laboured, vague thinking. At first, symptoms are concealed by memory aids, confabulation, etc. The mood is labile, shallow and blunted, and finally fatuous and euphoric. Judgement, self-control and initiative are all impaired. Sudden unpredictable and disproportionate reaction to frustration (the catastrophic reaction), organic orderliness and denial of illness are found. Psychological testing shows loss of normal perceptual ability (e.g. to distinguish figure and ground) and the presence of concrete thinking.

Atypical organic states

These are conditions which, instead of showing the usual organic symptoms listed above, mimic other mental illnesses, notably mania, depression and schizophrenia. Examples include the psychoses associated with addiction to amphetamine drugs, and the schizophreniform psychoses of epilepsy.

Differential diagnosis

If the examination suggested above has been carefully carried out there is usually little difficulty in distinguishing organic from functional states. Rarely, clouding of consciousness may be seen in acute mania and in acute schizophrenic excitement and give rise to difficulty. The only common source of difficulty is in puerperal psychosis where both symptomatic and functional psychoses may coexist.

Classification

Terms like 'delirium' and 'dementia' are descriptive. The following classification is based on aetiology.

Metabolic and nutritional disorders
1. Carbohydrate: functional and secondary hypoglycaemia
2. Vitamin deficiency:
   a. Aneurine hydrochloride (thiamine): Korsakoff's psychosis, Wernicke's encephalopathy
   b. Nicotinic acid: pellagra

c. Vitamin B_{12}: pernicious anaemia, 'megaloblastic madness'
3. Porphyrins: porphyria
4. Hormones:
   a. Thyroid: thyrotoxicosis, myxoedema
   b. Adrenal: Addison's disease, Cushing's syndrome
   c. Pituitary: Simmonds's disease
5. Oxygen:
   a. Anaesthesia
   b. Pulmonary disease
   c. Poor carrying power (carbon monoxide poisoning, anaemia).

Cerebro-vascular disorders
1. Cerebral atherosclerosis: 'arteriosclerotic dementia'
2. Slow cerebral blood flow: cardiac failure
3. Rarer vascular diseases: polyarteritis nodosa, disseminated lupus, temporal arteritis, thrombo-angiitis obliterans
4. Hypertensive encephalopathy.

Mechanical stresses
1. Space occupying lesions (primary and secondary tumour, abscess, etc.)
2. Trauma, acute and chronic (brain damage, sub-dural haematoma, post-concussional syndrome).

Infections
1. Meningitis
2. Encephalitis
3. Syphilis: general paralysis of the insane (G.P.I.)
4. Others, e.g. typhoid, cysticercosis, toxoplasmosis.

Intoxications
1. Exogenous
   a. Medication—e.g. reactions to sedatives, stimulants, chemotherapy, hormones, hypotensive drugs, antihistamines, antidepressants, steroids, digitalis
   b. Self-administered—alcohol, drugs, e.g. barbiturates, cannabis, L.S.D., etc.
   c. Occupational—lead, manganese, methyl chloride, carbon disulphide, etc.

2. Endogenous
   Renal failure; liver failure.

Degenerative disorders
1. Senile dementia.
2. Presenile dementia — simple, Huntington's chorea, Alzheimer's, Pick's and Jakob-Creutzfeld's diseases.

Epilepsy
Idiopathic and secondary, especially temporal lobe epilepsy.
Psychomotor attacks.
Post-ictal psychotic episodes (twilight states).
Epileptic dementia and personality change.

Clinical features

Alcohol
Delirium tremens. Usually occurs after intercurrent disease or sudden withdrawal of alcohol in a chronic addict. Clinically there is restlessness, insomnia and an affect of intense fear, with visual hallucinations, illusions and extreme distractibility. Coarse generalised tremor, tachycardia and excessive perspiration are typical. Treatment is by attention to fluid balance, sedation, vitamins.

Alcoholic dementia. There is gradual intellectual and moral deterioration. The affect is shallow and labile. Although socially pleasant, the patient is often domestically querulous and jealous. The process is arrested but not reversed by abstention.

Korsakoff's psychosis. A dysmnesic syndrome with disorientation, hallucinations, memory loss for recent events and disordered time sense. The patient compensates for his memory loss by describing fictitious events — *confabulation.* There is an associated peripheral neuritis.

Infections
General paralysis of the insane. Syphilis: symptoms occur on the average 10 years after the primary infection and the onset is between the ages of 30 and 45. Neurological examination shows dysarthria, tremor of face, lips and tongue, and Argyll-Robertson pupils. Later there may be spastic paralysis and epileptic fits.

Mental symptoms: there is an insidious deterioration of personality with an early loss of finer feelings. The patient becomes irritable, self-centred, less considerate of others and sexually and emotionally disinhibited. Recent memory is impaired. At this stage he may manage to cope with routine tasks but fails if judgement or initiative is required. There is depression or apathy and delusions of grandeur may develop. The disease, if untreated, proceeds to profound dementia and death.

Treatment is by penicillin and/or bismuth therapy. Ideally, by prevention: treating the primary infection.

Prognosis is good if diagnosed and treated early enough, although some personality defect will remain.

Fifty years ago one of the most common causes of dementia. Now rare because of treatment of primary infection and so diagnosis may be overlooked. May present with depression or simple dementia.

Encephalitis. In the acute stage there is delirium and there may be convulsions or neurological signs. In post-encephalitic states there is Parkinsonism, apathy and loss of initiative. In children marked personality and intellectual changes may follow the acute stage, resulting in aggressive and antisocial behaviour which may require institutional care. Milder degrees of personality change may also be found. The initial encephalitic illness may not have been severe and diagnosis is often missed. Serial antibody studies may clarify diagnosis.

Degenerative brain changes

Senile dementia. The symptoms are an exaggeration of the normal psychological changes of old age. These patients become narrow and restricted in outlook and memory is impaired. There is increasing difficulty in comprehension. Emotional expression is increased in the early stage and may lead to disturbed behaviour. Later there is blunting and poverty of emotion leading to apathy. The brain shows reduction in substance with neuronal degeneration and overgrowth of neuroglia. Treatment is symptomatic. The condition is progressive and death occurs within two to four years of the onset.

Arteriosclerotic dementia. All cerebral vessels from large arteries to capillaries show degenerative changes. Ischaemic changes are produced in the brain substance, e.g. cerebral softening and atrophy. Onset at a slightly younger age than in senile dementia. Memory loss is patchy and less general than in senile dementia and until the later stages the personality may be well preserved. At night these patients are often sleepless, restless and confused. The clinical picture is complicated in half of the cases by the effects of focal thrombosis, e.g. hemiplegia, dysphasia. The rate of deterioration varies and is erratic. Paranoid and depressive symptoms may accompany both senile and arteriosclerotic dementia, especially at the onset. Treatment is symptomatic.

Presenile dementia. Alzheimer's and Pick's diseases are relatively rare forms of cerebral degeneration occurring in the presenile period (45-60) and proceeding to complete dementia. Often apraxia and aphasia are prominent features.

Huntington's chorea is a familial hereditary disease inherited as an autosomal dominant. Age of onset 30-40 years. Early motor and mental changes may be observed. The motor inco-ordination is followed by early dementia.

Jakob-Creutzfeld disease is very rare. Dementia with ataxia, dysarthria and spasticity of the limbs. Death within two years. Recent work suggests possibility of slow-virus infection.

Trauma

Concussion. There is little demonstrable brain damage. Disturbance ranges from prolonged unconsciousness to mild clouding of consciousness.

Cerebral injury. Symptoms appear when concussion subsides, and vary with the site and extent of the damage. There may be intellectual changes which if mild are demonstrable only by special tests. Character change with loss of emotional inhibition may occur and euphoria and irritability are often marked. Recovery may take place up to many years after injury. Generally in head injury the duration of unconsciousness and of the retrograde amnesia are reliable guides to prognosis.

Space occupying lesions

Includes tumours (primary and secondary), subdural haematoma, cysts, etc. The usual symptoms are apathy, blunting of feeling and a reduction of alertness. There may be memory difficulty and impulsive behaviour. These symptoms are caused by the rise of intracranial pressure and have no localising value. Focal neurological signs may or may not be present. In some cases affective or schizophrenic illness may be mimicked.

Miscellaneous

In *myxoedema* there is apathy, retardation of thinking, poor memory and reduced intellectual ability. In addition the patient may be depressed or paranoid. *Thyrotoxicosis* may produce a mixture of anxiety, affective and organic symptoms. Mental symptoms may also occur in deficiency diseases, e.g. *pellagra,* and in chronic systematic diseases, e.g. evening delirium in *congestive heart failure* and euphoria in *multiple sclerosis.* Acute confusional symptoms or an 'hysterical' syndrome may occur in *porphyria.* In elderly patients minor degrees of physical illness (e.g. anaemia, chest or bladder infection, cardiac failure) may precipitate a confusional state. Toxic manifestations are also commonly associated with the use of sedatives and stimulant drugs. Barbiturates and amphetamines are particularly liable to cause confusion.

Confusion, excitement and sometimes hallucinations may be either idiosyncratic reactions or follow excessive dosage as in addiction. Some cases of amphetamine psychosis closely resemble acute paranoid schizophrenia.

Epilepsy

Epilepsy is the spontaneous paroxysmal discharge of excitation in the central nervous system. The resulting symptoms range from major convulsions with complete loss of consciousness to momentary tics with brief lapse of consciousness. Causal factors include neoplastic, hereditary, traumatic, infective and circulatory. Epilepsy is therefore not a disease entity but a symptom requiring investigation.

Incidence is difficult to assess because of the difficulty of establishing criteria, controlling age-factors, and of obtaining large-scale figures. A figure of 1/200 is generally accepted.

There are two main forms:

1. *Primary* or *idiopathic,* where the disturbance originates in the centrencephalic system

2. *Secondary* or *focal,* where the disturbance originates from a cortical focus and spreads to the centrencephalic system.

Clinical forms

Grand mal: 'major epilepsy' with definite loss of consciousness. The sequence is generally prodrome (e.g. irritability, restlessness), aura, convulsion, total loss of consciousness (with tonic spasm, followed by clonic jerkings). Disorientation, automatisms, explosive irritability, fugues, furor and twilight states may follow the fit.

Petit mal: 'minor epilepsy' with a characteristic 'absence' or transient loss of consciousness. Akinetic and myoclonic seizures may also occur. The patient is often unaware of the attack. Usually begins in childhood.

Psychical seizures. Forced thinking, déjà vu, hallucinations, illusions and perceptual anomalies are found in these attacks and are usually due to disturbance in the *temporal lobe,* as are:

Psychomotor attacks: partial loss of consciousness, semi-purposive movements. Masticatory movements are common. Twilight states with altered consciousness can be regarded as prolonged psychomotor attacks. Fugues may occur.

Reflex epilepsy: fits precipitated by sensory stimulation, e.g. music, bright colours, touch or flickering light (television).

Epileptic equivalents: emotional instability, compulsive actions, paroxysmal pains, 'thalamic' laughter, behaviour disorders are in rare cases akin to epileptic disorders.

Investigations

1. *History*
2. *Physical examination of the nervous system*
3. *Electroencephalography.* The EEG has contributed greatly to the study of epilepsy. Characteristic generalised spike and wave potentials, or focal spike potentials, may be noted. High amplitude dysrhythmic patterns of very fast and very slow activity may also be seen.

The EEG is a useful aid in investigating epilepsy, in indicating the existence of a focus and in assessing the need for further investigation and treatment. A normal record does not exclude epilepsy and the diagnosis ultimately rests on the history and observation of the seizure.

Treatment

1. Anticonvulsant medication. Phenobarbitone sodium B.P. 30 mg, t.i.d., increasing as necessary and sodium phenytoin B.P. (Epanutin) 50-100 mg, t.i.d., are suitable for the treatment of major seizures. Primidone B.P. (Mysoline) 250 mg, t.i.d., is especially useful in psychomotor epilepsy. Ethosuximide (250 mg capsules, 4-6 daily) and the dione derivatives (e.g. Troxidone caps B.P. 300 mg, 3-6 daily) are used in the management of petit mal attacks.

2. Advice on occupation and recreation, e.g. avoiding alcohol and risks such as driving or working near moving machinery.

3. Neurosurgery in certain cases of focal epilepsy.

Psychiatric aspects of epilepsy

Associated behaviour disorders and psychoses

In temporal lobe epilepsy, in addition to major seizures (in 50 per cent of cases), psychic and psychomotor attacks, there can be behaviour disturbance between the attacks. This is usually in the form of aggressive hostile behaviour, but paranoid, depressive and hysterical symptoms occur. In these cases the so-called *epileptic* personality may be seen. Such patients are self-centred, morose and religiose, and are pedantic and laborious both in speech and thought. Psychoses closely mimicking schizophrenia are seen in some cases. Temporal lobe epilepsy accounts for about one-third of all cases of epilepsy.

Epileptic dementia

In severe and uncontrolled epilepsy intellectual deterioration can occur over the years and lead to dementia. This must be distinguished from the temporary and reversible effects of seizures on memory (cf. ECT) and from the cumulative effects of large doses of anticonvulsants, especially phenobarbitone.

Psychological reactions to epilepsy

Although only a few show mental disturbances most

epileptics have psychological problems due to their illness and to society's attitude to the disorder, which is still regarded with superstition and fear. As it is not in their best interests to work machines or drive, epileptic patients have difficulties in finding employment and may become discouraged. Encouragement, help and interest are essential.

FURTHER READING

Talland, G. A. *Disorders of Memory and Learning*. Penguin.

7. Affective Disorders

The term affective disorder covers illnesses in which disturbance of affect (mood) is the primary symptom; all other symptoms are secondary. The mood may be persistently depressed or elated (in mania) and episodes of either type may occur in the same person, hence the term 'manic-depressive psychosis'. Illnesses with only one type of attack are called unipolar; with both manic and depressive episodes, bipolar.

Aetiology

Genetics. Twin studies show concordance rates of 70 per cent for monozygotic twins and 20 per cent for dizygotic twins. The incidence in the general population is 1 per cent and in first degree relatives 10-15 per cent. The type of transmission is probably polygenic, leading to varying degrees of predisposition. Bipolar and unipolar illnesses breed true.

Biochemistry. Inherited disorders must have biochemical origins. Various changes have been found in depressed patients, including increased adrenocortical activity and altered distribution of water and electrolytes, but the *monoamine theory* has provoked most research. There are three brain mono-amines — dopamine, noradrenaline and serotonin (5-hydroxytryptamine or 5 HT). The drug reserpine depletes the brain of mono-amines and may cause depression. There is evidence of altered 5 HT metabolism in depression. Some antidepressant drugs are mono-amine oxidase inhibitors (M.A.O.I.), and may work by increasing the concentration of mono-amines in the brain. The theory proposes that depression may be due to a decreased concentration of mono-amines at receptor sites in the brain.

Sex incidence. Affective illness is twice as common in women and is frequently associated with the puerperium and the menopause. Suicide and admission to hospital are more frequent premenstrually. During affective illness amenorrhoea often occurs. These factors suggest that an endocrine disturbance may be of aetiological importance.

Premorbid personality. Mild disturbances of mood are usual. Cyclothymic personalities are subject to mild swings of mood throughout life, unrelated to external causes. Depressive personalities are habitually gloomy, pessimistic and lacking in drive. Hypomanic personalities are habitually more cheerful, energetic and sociable than average.

Body build. Affective illness is often associated with the *pyknic body build,* stocky, round-faced, with thick short neck, fat trunk and slender extremities — the John Bull physique.

Age. The incidence rises with increasing age.

Seasonal influence. There is a higher incidence of affective illness and suicide in the late spring and early summer.

Social class. Affective illness is more frequent in the higher social classes.

Infection and drugs. Depressive illness often follows virus infections, particularly influenza and hepatitis, and may follow the administration of reserpine, methyldopa and steroids and oral contraceptives.

Childhood. Depressed patients have more often lost a parent in childhood than the rest of the population.

Loss. The usual precipitant of affective illness is the loss of a loved object. This may range from the serious (loss of spouse, employment, status, health, or self-respect) to the apparently trivial — loss of a pet.

Depression

Clinical picture

Psychological symptoms. There is a general loss of vitality which the patient may express as a loss of interest, or lack of energy. The patient appears tired and sad. Usually he withdraws from social activities and from people and his activity declines at work and in the home. The degree of depression can be slight or profound. Everything seems gloomy and hopeless. Anxiety may be present or the patient may try to conceal his symptoms ('smiling depression').

Diurnal variation. All symptoms tend to be worse in the early morning and improve as the day goes on.

Suicide. May be first sign of the illness. The risk of suicide is difficult to assess but is always present. Suicidal ideas should always be enquired about and taken seriously when elicited. Rarely, depressives may kill their relatives believing they must save them from a life of misery.

Retardation or slowing of thinking is usual, and is reflected in speech and movement. There is poverty of thought and difficulty in concentration. Rarely retardation can be severe enough to produce stupor. *Agitation* may be the dominant symptom in other cases, with obvious motor restlessness, pacing the floor and wringing of hands. There is accompanying anxiety, and speech is increased in amount but the content is repetitive, and poverty of thought remains.

Feelings of guilt are usual, with self-reproach and self-depreciation. In severe cases delusions may develop; the illness is regarded as a punishment for past sins, real or imagined. The patient may feel that he is despised and accused of sinfulness by others. There is self-absorption, hypochondriasis and hypochondriacal delusions may occur. There may also be delusions of poverty or 'nihilistic' delusions.

Hallucinations are rare but can occur in severe cases.

Depersonalisation and derealisation are not infrequent. The patient states that he has lost his feelings and has sensations of strangeness. He feels unreal and things look unreal to him. *Obsessional* thoughts and actions, usually with a content of guilt or self-blame, may be found.

Physical symptoms

Insomnia is usual. Typically the patient wakens early, but later both early and late insomnia and even total insomnia follow.

Anorexia, constipation, indigestion, weight loss, amenorrhoea and *loss of libido* are usual. Any of these may be the original presenting symptom. Hypochondriacal concern with such symptoms is common. Some depressions may present with unusual single symptoms, such as facial pain.

Summary

The typical symptoms of depression are loss of vitality, sadness, retardation, poverty of thought, self-depreciation, hopelessness, self-absorption, late insomnia and diurnal variation.

Types of depression

The symptoms described above are those of *endogenous* depression, i.e. depression arising from internal causes, genetic and biochemical. They respond to physical methods of treatment, and may run a bipolar course. *Neurotic (reactive) depressions* are twice as common but less clear-cut in their symptoms. They are usually less severe, related in time to a significant loss, and respond temporarily to reassurance, a change of environment or company. The typical sleep disturbance and diurnal variation of endogenous depression is rare and associated neurotic symptoms are common. They can be seen to stem from neurotic personality problems worsened or reactivated by obvious precipitants. They respond less well to physical treatment, and require psychotherapy.

The classification of depression has provoked much argument and research. One school of thought considers that the two types described are entirely different in quality, the other that the two patterns are at the extremes of a normal distribution curve with most patients falling between them. Whatever the truth, the two types described are valuable in predicting response to treatment.

Mania

Clinical picture

Mania is rarer than depression. The patient feels perfectly well physically and mentally and is usually brought to the doctor by his family. The mood is euphoric, with flashes of irritability, and varies from mild elation to wild hilarity and excitement. The patient's cheerfulness is infectious but quickly becomes tiresome. There is increased mental and physical activity; less sleep is required and there is talkativeness and over-optimistic planning for the future. The patient is tactless and disinhibited, and may be promiscuous and extravagant.

Thinking. The stream of thought is rapid but rarely to the point. Thinking is not directed logically but by casual association, e.g. sounds, puns, rhymes (flight of ideas).

Attention cannot be sustained for any time.

Delusions when present are usually grandiose and unsustained. Severe cases may be *disorientated* and *restless* so that physical exhaustion may be a risk to life.

Course and prognosis

Affective disorders are common. In a 10 year period in general practice about 1 in every 10 of the practice population will complain of depression. About ten cases of depression are seen for each one of mania.

The typical attack lasts from 6 to 9 months but may range from hours to many years. Complete recovery from the attack is the rule but some 10 per cent become chronic, with permanent or fluctuating mood changes. In depression two-thirds of patients have a single attack, in mania one-half never have a recurrence. In patients who have recurrent attacks most will have repeated attacks of depression, about one in three will be bipolar (both manic and depressive) and only 4 per cent will have repeated attacks of mania. The intervals are irregular and unpredictable, but with increasing number of attacks the time interval tends to diminish.

Favourable prognostic features and indicators of good response to physical treatment include typical endogenous symptoms, an abrupt onset, a stable premorbid personality without neurotic traits, and paradoxically, severity of the attack. Unfavourable features include depersonalisation, hypochondriasis, hysterical traits and atypical symptoms of any kind.

Differential diagnosis

Complaints of depression are made in many illnesses. Organic states, especially cerebral tumour and arterio-sclerosis, may present with depressive symptoms. In adolescents or young adults depression may be an early symptom of schizophrenia.

The diagnosis of depression may be missed, thereby increasing the risk of suicide. In early cases of depression with predominant anxiety a neurotic illness may be diagnosed. When the presenting symptoms of depression are physical (anorexia, weight loss, loss of libido, etc.) extensive physical investigations may be made and the correct diagnosis delayed.

Hypomania must be differentiated from the effects of stimulant drugs, alcohol, catatonic excitement and the euphoric picture associated with frontal lobe lesions.

Treatment

Electro-convulsive therapy produces remission in over 80 per cent of severe depressions. Antidepressant drugs benefit over 60 per cent of cases but side effects can be troublesome and the delay in response for 2 to 4 weeks is worrying in potentially suicidal patients. ECT and antidepressant drugs are often used in combination. Phenothiazines are used in large doses to control manic symptoms.

These treatments do not prevent further attacks. Long term maintenance treatment with lithium preparations diminishes the frequency and severity of both manic and depressive episodes.

See notes on treatment (p. 112-14).

8. Schizophrenia

Schizophrenia is the most severe form of functional psychosis producing the greatest disorganisation of personality. In severe cases the patient is out of contact with reality to such an extent that his ideas and behaviour are patently abnormal. The illness typically runs a gradual course towards chronicity but may occur in attacks. Complete spontaneous recovery is rare and the untreated disease usually 'burns out' after some years leaving a dilapidated personality — the 'defect state'. The condition was first delineated in 1896 on the basis of its symptoms and natural history by Kraepelin, who used the label dementia praecox. In 1911 Bleuler coined the name schizophrenia to mark the 'splitting' or disruption of psychic function which characterises the illness. There are international differences in diagnostic criteria, especially between Europe and the U.S.A., and many psychiatrists now speak of the 'schizophrenias' as a group of related disorders.

Statistics

The estimated risk of schizophrenia at some time in life is 0.5-1 per cent. Schizophrenia accounts for some 15 per cent of admissions to psychiatric hospitals, for 45 per cent of the hospital population, and the majority of long-stay patients. The disease is more common in males than females and most cases begin before the age of 30.

Symptomatology

A wide range of symptoms occurs in various combinations and at different stages in the course of the disorder. Some are found in other conditions, some are almost confined to schizophrenia and are of greater diagnostic significance.

Disorder of thought
This refers to the form rather than the content: formal

thought disorder. Thinking is woolly and diffuse. The normal associations between ideas are disrupted ('knight's move' thinking). The patient may experience sudden halts in his thinking (thought blocking). Concrete thinking (inability to think in abstract terms) may be demonstrated by asking the patient to give the general meaning of well-known proverbs. Reasoning is disturbed by the intrusion of personal themes (autistic or dereistic thinking), and by inability to select ideas (overinclusive thinking).

Disorder of emotion

The emotional reaction and mood are inappropriate, or incongruous with the patient's situation or thoughts. Later blunting and apathy develop. An early sign is a lack of rapport found at interview.

Disorder of volition

There is loss of will-power, lassitude and lack of drive, often shown by a falling-off in housework, studying and work. At times excessive obstinacy, negativism or automatic obedience may be found.

Catatonia

Abnormality of movement may occur with awkward, poorly co-ordinated movements and gait, grimacing, posturing and, in extreme cases, waxy flexibility and echopraxia.

Hallucinations

These occur in many illnesses but in schizophrenia are found in a setting of clear consciousness. They are usually auditory, but other sensory modalities may be involved.

Delusions

Primary delusions: the sudden appearance of a fully developed delusion from a normal perception which the patient instantly accepts as overwhelmingly convincing.

Secondary delusions are false beliefs arising from other symptoms, e.g. the patient may 'explain' thought disorder by coming to believe that thoughts are being put into his head by an outside agency, or that his thoughts are being interfered with.

Disturbances of expression

Thought disorder and hallucinations are often reflected in

speech (neologisms, word salad), mannered handwriting, and unusual paintings and poems.

Withdrawal

As a result of the above symptoms, withdrawal from normal social contacts and activities is often an early symptom.

Diagnosis

Negative findings are important. Manic or depressive symptoms, or a previous history of them, should be absent. There should be no history of alcohol or drug abuse which might account for the symptoms. Consciousness must be clear, memory and orientation intact. If delusions or hallucinations are not present, convincing thought disorder must be demonstrated. Epilepsy must be excluded.

Schizophrenia can then be diagnosed with confidence if several of Schneider's *first rank symptoms* can be elicited. These comprise of the experiences of thought insertion, thought withdrawal and thought broadcasting; feelings of passivity (i.e. the experience of sensations, emotions or even movements being caused or controlled by an outside agency); voices heard talking about the patient in the third person, voices giving a running commentary on the patient's thoughts or behaviour, voices heard to be voicing the patient's own thoughts; and lastly, primary delusions.

In many early cases the diagnosis is doubtful. The premorbid personality and family history may give supporting evidence, but often the progress of the condition must be observed for some time to clarify the diagnosis.

Clinical picture

The following subtypes of schizophrenia are not separate clinical entities but are convenient methods of classifying schizophrenic reactions.

Hebephrenic schizophrenia. The onset is usually in the late teens. Early symptoms are perplexity, poor concentration, vagueness, day-dreaming, self-consciousness, moodiness, depression, apathy, transient delusions, indiscriminate concern with pseudo-scientific and pseudo-philosophical ideas, feelings of inferiority and inadequancy. Thought disturbance becomes obvious and there may be concrete thinking or thought blocking. Emotional incongruity is characteristic.

Paranoid schizophrenia. The typical symptoms are primary and secondary delusions of persecution with auditory hallucinations. The onset is later than in hebephrenic schizophrenia, usually between 30 and 50 years. The course is chronic with minimal deterioration of personality. Misinterpretations of the actions of others may be incorporated in ideas of persecution. The delusions may be 'encapsulated' and the patient may behave normally, but usually his delusional ideas bring him into conflict with society. Although the illness takes a chronic course, there may be periodic fluctuation in the symptoms. The florid illness is often preceded by paranoid traits of personality — hypersensitive or self-conscious individuals who take offence at harmless remarks or who are isolated by reason of deformity, deafness, language difficulty, etc.

Catatonic schizophrenia. Stereotyped behaviour, negativism, posturing, immobility and stupor are the most obvious characteristics. Thought blocking, neologisms, hallucinations may also occur. Acute excitement may be the first sign of the disease. Catatonic symptoms have become increasingly rare in the last 30 years: many may have been a product of institutional neurosis (see p. 106).

Simple schizophrenia. As there are no florid features the diagnosis may be missed for many years. The onset, usually during adolescence, is insidious and the course very slowly progressive. Many cases never reach hospital. Primary symptoms of emotional blunting, loss of volition and thought disorder are usual. The patients drift through life and are solitary; their social level sinks and they may drift into poverty, petty crime, prostitution and vagrancy.

Aetiology

The cause of schizophrenia is unknown and represents one of the greatest research challenges of contemporary medicine. Much research has already been done and many predisposing and precipitating factors are known.

Heredity. The importance of genetic factors has been

convincingly demonstrated. The risk in the general population is 1 per cent, in parents of schizophrenics 5 per cent, in siblings 8 per cent and in children 10 per cent. This last figure persists even when the children have been separated from the parent from birth. The concordance in monozygotic twins is 30-40 per cent.

Environment. These twin figures suggest that environmental factors must play some part in the appearance of the disease in predisposed individuals. Some workers (Laing, Goffman) suggest that schizophrenia is not a disease but a response to intolerable emotional pressures in the family and society, but such extreme views, although fashionable with the public, lack experimental support. Much careful work on childhood influences, particularly on the personalities of the parents, is inconclusive. It has been shown that stresses such as promotion or bereavement are more common in the month preceding the onset or relapses.

Premorbid personality. The previous personality of the patient is often 'schizoid'. This solitary and withdrawn behaviour may explain the large number of single schizophrenics.

Physique. Many schizophrenics are of asthenic build and in the established case there may be poor peripheral circulation, cold cyanotic extremities, and amenorrhoea.

Biochemistry. Phantasticant drugs and addiction to amphetamine produce symptoms akin to schizophrenia. The chemical structure of these drugs led to much research on adrenaline and serotonin with inconclusive results. Numerous minor defects of metabolism have been found. In periodic catatonia, a rare condition, nitrogen retention occurs.

Immunology. There is current interest in the role of brain antibodies in the genesis of schizophrenia.

Course and prognosis

Schizophrenia is not fatal except through suicide. The general trend is towards disintegration of the personality, but the process may be arrested at any point, leaving a personality defect which may be inconspicuous or obvious. The remission rate without treatment was about 20 per cent, but with treatment some two-thirds make a social recovery. In the past two-thirds of schizophrenics spent their lives in hospital, today fewer than one in ten require permanent hospital care.

Favourable prognostic factors include absence of family history of the disease, normal personality, and stable family background and work record. Features of the illness associated with a good outcome include acute onset, obvious precipitants, retention of normal emotional response, presence of catatonic symptoms, retention of drive and initiative. Early treatment favours a favourable outcome.

Differential diagnosis

Schizophrenia must be distinguished from:

1. Psychological difficulties of *normal adolescence*. This may be especially difficult in shy, sensitive and highly intelligent students.

2. *Symptomatic schizophrenia*. In several conditions, notably psychoses associated with temporal-lobe epilepsy and amphetamine addiction, the symptoms may be indistinguishable from those of schizophrenia.

3. *Affective psychoses*. Some atypical depressions or manias may give rise to diagnostic difficulty. When doubt exists and affective symptoms are prominent the term *schizo-affective psychosis* is sometimes used.

4. Paranoid psychosis produced by *alcoholism,* or the early symptoms of an *organic dementia* may mimic schizophrenia.

Treatment

In the acute phase phenothiazine drugs are given in large doses, often with ECT. Phenothiazines are effective in reducing delusions, hallucinations and disturbed thinking and behaviour, but less effective in altering negative symptoms such as emotional blunting and loss of volition. Maintenance therapy must be given over years and relapse rates are high when attempts are made to stop drugs. As many patients fail to take oral medication regularly, long acting preprarations (e.g. fluphenazine decanoate) given every two to four weeks are widely used.

Social therapy is necessary. Schizophrenics require intensive rehabilitation, social and industrial, but the amount of stimulation must be matched to individual requirements. Excessive stimulation has been shown to lead to relapse, too little to continuing withdrawal and chronicity. Rehabilitation must be planned, sometimes over several years, and involves the services of nurses, social workers, occupational therapists and recreational therapists. A variety of facilities is also necessary, ranging from night wards, day hospitals and industrial therapy units to lengthy courses of training in rehabilitation units, and hostel accommodation in the community.

FURTHER READING

Boyers R. (Ed.) *Laing and Anti-Psychiatry*. Penguin.
Clark, D. *Administrative Therapy*. Penguin.
Laing, R. D. *The Divided Self*. Penguin.

9. Personality Disorder and Psychopathy

There is great variety in human personality; some people are more irritable, some tidier than others, and so on. Some whose personalities deviate markedly from the average may suffer by being unusual, make others suffer, or both. Such individuals are not ill, but their disordered personality may bring them to the attention of doctors and social agencies or into conflict with society and the law.

The many labels that are attached to this group by psychiatrists reflect the unsatisfactory state of classification. The term 'moral insanity' was first used by Pritchard in 1835 to describe 'persons of a singular, wayward and eccentric character'. Other terms which have been used include neurotic character, character disorder, sociopathy and psychopathic personality. The International Statistical Classification of Diseases favours 'personality disorder' with various sub-divisions, and this usage is followed here. As their names suggest, most of the varieties have associations with psychiatric disorders: a particular disorder of personality may predispose to a particular neurosis or psychosis.

Varieties of personality disorder

Cyclothymic (affective): people who are persistently gloomy and persistently optimistic, or who alternative between these extremes; they are prone to develop affective illnesses (see Chap. 7).

Schizoid: individuals who are introverted and withdrawn. Because of their shy, aloof and reserved manner they have few friends and are by nature solitary. They may show odd and eccentric behaviour. Common precursor of schizophrenia and frequent in the relatives of schizophrenics.

Paranoid: personalities who make excessive use of projection as a defence mechanism — they blame others to excess. They may be sensitive and downtrodden, blaming others for their lack of success in life; or they may be aggressive, suspicious and irritable individuals, ever ready to take offence, and sometimes resorting to litigation in defence of over-valued ideas.

Hysterical (see p. 55).

Obsessional (anankastic) (see p. 56).

Antisocial or psychopathic personality. This description is applied to individuals who behave in a seriously antisocial way, showing a wide range of repetitive antisocial behaviour. They do not appear to learn from experience or punishment. They are usually impulsive, irresponsible and aggressive. They show little feeling for others and their cold callous personality sets them apart from other criminals who readily recognise them as abnormal. These individuals frequently have accompanying neurotic symptoms and a history of parasuicide. There is a family history of antisocial behaviour and alcoholism. The vast majority have a history of antisocial behaviour in childhood with episodes of truancy, serious disobedience and theft. The majority show some maturation in personality and improvement in their behaviour between the age of 30 and 40 years. Only a minority of aggressive criminals and murderers fall into this category (see also Chap. 19).

10. The Psychoneuroses

Psychoneurotic disorders, commonly referred to as 'nervous' illnesses, are characterised by disturbances of feelings, attitudes and habits severe enough to impair the patient's life or to reduce his efficiency. The symptoms are best understood as manifestations of anxiety or as ineffective ways of dealing with anxiety.

Incidence: high, but difficult to estimate accurately. This group of disorders is probably the commonest single cause of ill health encountered in general practice. Symptoms of anxiety and depression are frequent, hysterical and obsessional symptoms less so.

Classification. The psychoneuroses are classified by the symptoms. Overlap occurs between the various subdivisions and many mixed types of psychoneurosis occur, e.g. anxiety and hysterical symptoms may co-exist.

Anxiety neurosis

Anxiety is a fundamental mode of response experienced by everyone. It is analogous to pain in that both serve as a warning to the organism. In psychoneurosis anxiety appears inappropriate to the situation or excessive in degree.

In anxiety neurosis patients show signs of increased autonomic activity, both sympathetic and parasympathetic. There are feelings of tension, concern, apprehension, difficulty in concentrating and insomnia, combined with palpitations, sweating, gastric disturbance, restlessness, tremulousness, 'tension headache', diarrhoea. The symptoms may be persistent or take the form of acute attacks of anxiety lasting a few minutes or several hours. Depressive symptoms or symptoms of fatigue ('neurasthenia') are often associated with anxiety.

Acute anxiety states occurring in previously stable personalities are usually short-lived and have a good prognosis. Chronic and recurrent anxiety states are found in *anxious personalities,* who have always been timid, diffident, indecisive, fearful and worrying.

Phobic states

A phobia is an unreasonable fear, out of proportion to the situation, which cannot be voluntarily controlled and which leads to avoidance of the object or feared situation. Fears may be normal or abnormal, the dividing line often being a question of severity and incapacity, e.g. fears of flying, of spiders, and of heights. Abnormal fears can be divided into fears of external and internal stimuli. Phobias of internal stimuli comprise obsessive phobias (see obsessional neurosis) and illness phobias (hypochondriasis, venereophobia, etc.). Most fears are of external stimuli. Two-thirds show agoraphobia, and the remainder social phobias, or specific phobias, especially of animals.

Agoraphobia ('housebound housewife' syndrome)

Agoraphobia is the commonest phobic disorder, and one of the most common neuroses in women, who make up 75 per cent of patients. Usually begins in young adult life. Literally a fear of the *agora* (the Greek place of assembly or marketplace). The patient fears going out alone, social situations, shopping, travelling, and confined spaces, such as cinemas and churches. There is associated general anxiety, panic attacks, feelings of dizziness and unsteadiness, and often depression or depersonalisation. If the condition becomes established and lasts for more than a year it tends to run a chronic fluctuating course. The husband becomes involved in doing a great deal for his wife, and after a time there is considerable secondary gain to the patient. Often agoraphobic patients do well in hospital but relapse rapidly on returning home.

Social phobias

The next most common group of phobias. Again common in young adults and more frequent in women, usually with shy, sensitive personalities. The fear of social situations may be general but often is concerned with one particular social situation — eating or drinking in public, writing or speaking, or using public toilets. There is little general anxiety.

Hysteria

The symptoms of hysteria usually solve a conflict and resolve the associated anxiety. They have a *motivation* which is unrecognised by the patient and is therefore unconscious. Once established the symptom may provide gain to the patient. Symptoms which are feigned, i.e. consciously produced, are found in malingering, which can usually be distinguished from hysteria. The features of the *hysterical personality* are sometimes present before symptoms develop. Such personalities are dramatic, scene-loving and attention craving, emotionally shallow and insincere, sexually titillating but basically frigid. They tend to manipulate their families and friends and can be recognised by their provocative manner and dress and by their dramatic gestures and extravagant use of language. Hysterical patients have often experienced periods of illness in childhood and have learned that sickness can be 'rewarding' in gaining sympathy and attention.

In *conversion* hysteria the conflict is solved by the development of a somatic symptom, e.g. paralysis, anaesthesia, blindness. The symptoms are varied and may mimic any physical illness. Diagnosis may be complicated when hysterical symptoms and physical illness coexist and thorough investigation and observation are needed in all cases. Physical illness must be excluded, but to make the diagnosis of hysteria it is also necessary to show that the symptom serves a purpose, is meaningful or produces gain for the patient. When re-examined after some years many patients, confidently diagnosed as having hysteria by neurologists or psychiatrists, have developed a variety of organic diseases.

In *dissociative* reactions particular experiences or situations are dissociated from consciousness and the patient shows amnesia, a fugue state, somnambulism or very rarely multiple personality. So called 'hysterical' fits are rare, and usually prove to be temporal lobe seizures. Part of the dissociation in all hysterical reactions is illustrated by the hysteric's bland cheerful attitude to his symptoms ('belle indifference').

The prognosis for isolated and recently acquired hysterical

symptoms is favourable. Psychotherapy and procedures using suggestion, such as hypnosis and abreaction, are usually employed. When the patient's gain from his symptom is considerable, environmental manipulation may be necessary. When hysterical personality traits are marked further hysterical symptoms can be anticipated as a reaction to future conflicts and stresses. The symptoms of hysteria vary in different cultures and epochs. The 'stocking' anaesthesias and paraplegias which were frequent in the 19th century are rarely seen today and more indefinite and less easily diagnosed complaints are the rule.

Obsessional neurosis

An *obsession* exists whenever a person cannot exclude thoughts from consciousness, distinguishes them as unreasonable and attempts to resist them but cannot do so. Obsessions occur in many psychiatric conditions, notably in depressive illness and schizophrenia. When they are primary the diagnosis of obsessive compulsive or obsessive ruminative neurosis is made. *Rumination* is the term applied to repetitive obsessional thinking; *compulsions* are acts which the patient feels compelled to carry out. When these acts are stereotyped and repetitive they become rituals. Obsessions with sex, violence, death, dirt, excrement and germs are usual. Washing and checking rituals are common.

Obsessional neurosis is often associated with an *obsessional personality* in which there is a tendency to excessive orderliness, punctuality, scrupulousness and rigidity of behaviour and attitudes.

The incidence of obsessional neurosis is low. Age of onset is usually between 15 and 25. These neuroses, when fully developed, have a poorer prognosis than other neurotic reactions and are resistant to treatment. Clomipramine, orally or by infusion, may be of value. Intensive psychotherapy is rarely indicated but supportive psychotherapy is helpful. In very severe and chronic cases pre-frontal leucotomy is of value and behaviour therapy is also useful.

Post-traumatic neurosis

This type of psychoneurosis is seen in patients who have

been subjected to a trauma which has involved a sudden threat to life. Physical injury may or may not occur. Most cases occur after accidents and claims for compensation often complicate diagnosis and treatment to the extent that *accident neurosis* or *compensation neurosis* have become alternative labels for the condition. In *battle neurosis* the strain and exhaustion of combat, with or without a traumatic incident, initiates symptoms.

The symptoms may comprise any of the neurotic symptoms already mentioned but irritability, tension, poor concentration and nightmares, often of a repetitive kind, are common. Motor manifestations, especially tics, may occur.

The prognosis is generally good. Post-traumatic neurosis is common after head injury and these cases have a poorer prognosis, particularly when there is a claim for compensation.

Aetiology of psychoneurosis

Psychoneurotic reactions arise from the interaction of the patient's make-up and his current problems and stresses. The patient's make-up combines past experience (especially in childhood) and genetic constitution. In some neurotic reactions, e.g. traumatic neurosis, past experience and constitution are of little importance and current problems and stresses paramount; in the majority, constitution and early experience are more important than current problems which act only as precipitants. The form of illness is generally related to the basic personality of the individual (e.g. anxious, obsessional, hysterical). The symptoms of psychoneurosis can be regarded as ineffectual means of dealing with emotional conflict.

Superficially the symptoms of neurosis seem to be inappropriate or exaggerated responses by the patient to his current life situation. This is because the causes are 'intrapsychic', i.e. stem from past experiences and attitudes. 'Intrapsychic anxiety' may be expressed directly, or other neurotic symptoms may be developed to deal with such anxiety.

This theory derives from Freud, and is applied to the main

types of psychoneurosis as follows:

Anxiety neurosis. The anxiety from intrapsychic conflicts is released directly as anxiety symptoms.

Phobic anxiety state. The phobia concentrates anxiety to specific situations and the patient is left free to cope with other situations without difficulty.

Hysteria. The patient solves a conflict by producing a somatic symptom. The symptom can often be viewed as a symbolic representation of the conflict in that it combines the expression of an unconscious wish with the arousal of defences against that wish (e.g. desire to run away and fear of being thought a coward 'solved' by production of hysterical paralysis).

Obsessional neurosis. The symptoms represent a defence against instinctual impulses, often of an aggressive nature. The psychodynamic formulation emphasises the importance of guilt resulting from such impulses and sees the rituals and obsessions as attempts to undo or isolate this guilt. The obsessional neurotic shows in an exaggerated and distorted form the characteristics of the obsessional personality (anal-erotic character), namely the need to achieve security by arranging the environment in an ordered regular fashion, which Freud regarded as a reaction to toilet training.

Treatment of psychoneurosis

Psychological treatment (see p. 103) has its main application in the psychoneuroses. Sedatives and tranquillisers (see p. 110) are widely prescribed as symptomatic treatment. Barbiturates are a most effective remedy for anxiety but carry serious risks of habituation and addiction. Tranquillising drugs are less addictive and some (e.g. chlordiazepoxide, diazepam) are equally effective.

FURTHER READING

Kraupl-Taylor, F. (1966) *Psychopathology.* Butterworths.
Lowe, G. R., *Personal Relationships in Psychological Disorders.* Penguin.

11. Alcoholism

The World Health Organisation attempted to define alcoholics as 'those excessive drinkers whose dependence on alcohol has attained such a degree that it causes a noticable mental disturbance or an interference with their bodily and mental health, their interpersonal relations and their smooth social and economic functioning'.

This is a social rather than a medical definition and depends on social and cultural factors which may vary, e.g. excessive for whom, when, compared with what other group, in what culture? It is generally agreed that alcoholism is a *dependency disorder,* in which the alcoholic shows both psychological and physical dependence. Physical dependence implies that withdrawal leads to a characteristic syndrome, and this holds true for established drinking. It can easily be seen how psychological dependence, produced by the anxiety-relieving effects of alcohol, can in time lead to physical dependence.

Aetiology

A plausible theory must explain why the majority of the population drinks alcohol but only a minority becomes dependent. It must also explain other known facts about alcoholism. Male cases outnumber women by at least five to one. Many are single, and the peak age of presentation is from 40 to 50 years. It is more common at the extremes of social class. There are racial and national differences: Scots outnumber English, Catholics usually outnumber Jews, and blacks outnumber whites in the U.S.A. Rural rates are higher than urban, and those in the drink trade or involved in business entertaining have higher rates. The sons of alcoholics have twice the normal risk.

Much research — genetic, social, metabolic, endocrine, and psychological — has yielded no convincing results. Learning theory offers a simple theory of the development of alcoholism in terms of operant conditioning; immediate rewards (relief) are more effective than delayed punishment (hangover). Later, non-reward factors (fear of withdrawal symptoms) may reinforce continued drinking.

Prevalence

Prevalence is about 1 per cent in Britain, but concealment and denial make accurate figures impossible to obtain. First admission rates for alcoholism underestimate the problem. Jellinek devised a formula for estimating prevalence from deaths due to alcoholic cirrhosis which proved reasonably accurate. Consumption of spirits, beer and wine is rising in Britain, and alcoholism is also rising, especially in younger males.

Types

1. Loss of control. Bout drinking; one drink triggers off a binge. Usually spirits. Commonest in Britain and North America.
2. Inability to abstain. Constant daily drinking, usually of wine or beer. Common in Italy and France.

Stages

1. Symptomatic pre-dependent.
2. Prodromal. The drinker avoids discussing his consumption, begins secret drinking, minimises amount, feels guilty, and may have amnesia for the previous night's drinking (alcoholic palimpsests).
3. Dependency. Psychological and physical — withdrawal signs if stops.
4. Chronic. Social deterioration, physical and psychiatric complications.

Diagnosis

Many alcoholics deny difficulties and are brought reluctantly by relatives. They may agree that they have a drinking problem but argue about the label of alcoholism, which should be avoided. Enquire about work and domestic problems, withdrawal symptoms, amnesia, morning shakiness, nausea. Obtain account from relative.

Complications

Social

By the time the alcoholic is willing to accept help these are almost inevitable. Frequent changes of job or unemployment, unhappy marriage or divorce, financial and housing problems, multiple and complicated financial difficulties.

Physical

1. Acute intoxication, coma, etc.
2. Withdrawal syndromes: the 'shakes', delirium tremens.
3. Deficiency and nutritional syndromes: peripheral neuropathy, Korsakov's psychosis, Wernicke's encephalopathy (confusion, ataxia, eye signs — nystagmus, rectus palsy).
4. Epilepsy: common at various stages of alcoholism.
5. Other complications include myopathies, cardiac disease, cirrhosis, pancreatic disease, malabsorption disorders, hypoglycaemia, hyperlipaemia, magnesium deficiency.

Psychiatric

1. Alcoholic hallucinosis
2. Alcoholic paranoid state — often 'morbid jealousy syndrome'
3. Alcoholic dementia.
4. Suicide.

Treatment and prognosis

Prognosis is poor — even those who do well usually have initial relapses. At best one-third remain abstinent, one-third are unchanged, and one-third deteriorate. There is no evidence that admission is superior to out-patient treatment. Sedatives and psychotropic drugs are best avoided in the long-term, as they are likely to be abused. Treatments include Antabuse (disulfiram), Abstem (citrated calcium carbide), aversion therapy with apomorphine or electric shock and, most successful, group methods, notably Alcoholics Anonymous.

After-care hostels are being developed. Understandably the alcoholic encounters much distrust and prejudice during rehabilitation. The patient who refuses help often accepts it when his condition has deteriorated. Many doctors take a moralistic attitude to alcoholism, or fail to diagnose it in the early stages.

FURTHER READING

Kessel, N. & Walton, H. *Alcoholism*. Penguin.

12. Drug Dependence

The World Health Organisation has defined drug dependence as a 'state of periodic or chronic intoxication, detrimental to the individual and to society, produced by the repeated consumption of the drug. Its characteristics include: an overpowering desire or need to continue taking the drug and to obtain it by any means; a tendency to increase the dose; psychic and sometimes physical dependence on the effects of the drug.'

For many years dependence on dangerous drugs was rare in the United Kingdom and occurred mainly in professional workers with access to drugs (e.g. doctors, pharmacists, nurses) or was iatrogenic, following the prescription of powerful analgesics post-operatively or in chronic physical illness. These cases have been overshadowed in the last decade by an alarming increase in addiction in young people. Drugs used by addicts include morphine, cocaine, synthetic analgesics (pethidine, physeptone), barbiturates and amphetamines. The use of marihuana (hashish) is increasing among young people but its status as a true drug of addiction and as a precursor of abuse of 'hard' drugs is debatable.

Morphine, heroin (Di-acetyl-morphine)

Subcutaneous ('skin-pop') and intravenous ('main-line') routes are used. Nausea, sweating and malaise occur before pleasurable 'honeymoon stage'. Light sleep and wakefulness alternate allowing the 'opium dreams' to occur. Constipation and pupillary contraction are found. Appetite is poor and libido is reduced. Abstinence syndrome occurs 9-12 hours after withdrawal — perspiration, yawning, restlessness, insomnia, rhinorrhoea, rigor, diarrhoea and cramps.

Cocaine

Uncommon by itself but often taken with other drugs to increase libido. Drugs are sniffed in 'decks' with the risk of nasal septal perforation, or are taken by 'main-line'. Initial alertness and increased energy are often followed by collapse, cramps, twitching, delirium or toxic psychosis. Formication (tactile hallucinations) occurs.

Pethidine

Highest incidence in doctors and nurses who may take it for relief of pain (e.g. dysmenorrhoea). Muscular twitching, tremor, dilated pupils, confusion and fits may be found. EEG changes occur.

Barbiturates

Common in United States of America and Western Europe. May alternate with amphetamine taking. Severe dependence when about 0·8g or more are taken each day. Confusion and ataxia or nystagmus is common and may simulate dementia, drunkenness or neurological lesion. Abrupt withdrawal usually produces convulsions. Withdrawal symptoms are anxiety, headache, tremor, vomiting and weakness.

Amphetamines

Commenced with the prescription of this and related drugs (e.g. phenmetrazine) to curb appetite. Initial stimulation is followed by toxic effects of the drug and paranoid psychosis mimicking schizophrenia may be seen. Main withdrawal symptom is depression. In many areas doctors have agreed to ban prescription of amphetamine and related drugs.

Lysergic acid diethylamide 25 (LSD 25)

May be used to produce hallucinations and pseudomystical experiences. Danger of precipitating schizophrenia-like psychosis. True addiction unlikely.

Cannabis, marihuana

World wide increase in use of this drug (grass, pot, ganja, reefer, hash, etc.) by younger people. Feared by many authorities as leading to other drugs ('escalation') but occasional use is probably safe. Drug is illegal in most countries and may be used as part of protest against authority. Effects erratic but usually dreamy, tranquil state, increased auditory sensibility, sexual excitement. Not unlike effects of alcohol. Dangerous when driving.

Glue sniffing

A number of organic solvents are abused by young people, often the very young. All are potentially dangerous and permanent damage to the brain, liver and kidney may result.

Treatment

The Dangerous Drugs Regulations, 1968 lay down that heroin and cocaine, apart from their analgesic use, may be prescribed only by doctors specially licensed by the Home Secretary. In practice such doctors are usually hospital consultants who treat heroin addiction. The Government has powers to introduce further regulations limiting prescribing of dangerous drugs at any time it may prove necessary. There is a statutory requirement for any doctor seeing an addict to send written particulars to the Home Office within seven days. Licences are only valid for prescribing at a named hospital, such departments becoming 'special centres'.

These regulations were designed to make heroin available to registered addicts and minimise the growth of a 'black-market'. The lack of compulsion means that many addicts seek maintenance supplies rather than cure. For withdrawal admission to hospital is essential and methadone and chlorpromazine are used. Extensive psychotherapy and rehabilitation are essential. The mortality from intercurrent infection among addicts, e.g. serum hepatitis, septicaemia, is high and the prognosis poor.

FURTHER READING

The Non-Medical Use of Drugs, Interim report of the Canadian Government's commission of inquiry. Penguin.
Wells, B. *Psychedelic Drugs*. Penguin.

13. Disorders of Sex and Reproduction

Because of the attitudes of society and of individuals it is difficult to build up an adequate body of knowledge of human sexual behaviour. Paradoxically, more is known about sexual deviations than about normal sexuality.

To deal with the sexual problems brought by patients the doctor should be able to relate them to the available systematic knowledge rather than to his own prejudices, moral attitudes and limited personal experience. Ethical and religious considerations are involved in sexual behaviour and should always be respected. The doctor's task is to understand and not to pass judgement.

In all animals sexual drives stem from the reproductive instinct but in humans because of the long period of maturation the emotional concomitants are of particular importance. Physical sexual maturity is reached in adolescence. Psychosexual maturity, involving stable sexual adjustment and stable and lasting emotional relationships is only reached later and in a few people it is never fully attained.

The child's attitude to his parents and his emotional relationships with them have an important effect in determining adult sexual behaviour, e.g. the young man tends to choose girl-friends according to the ideas of femininity which he has built up from his contacts with his mother. The Freudian theory of infantile sexuality, culminating in the 'Oedipal situation', lays particular stress on these factors in personality and psychosexual development.

Adolescence

Sexual problems are universal at this time and medical advice is often sought. The adolescent though sexually mature is psychologically immature and unable to take on adult responsibilities, at least in Western civilisation. The resulting conflict leads to anxiety and a search for sexual outlets.

Masturbation as an outlet for adolescents is normal. Guilt feelings are often aroused, however, and are fostered by folklore and rumours suggesting that masturbation does physical, mental and moral damage. With psychosexual maturity and heterosexual activity, masturbation is reduced.

Homosexual behaviour, i.e. sexual activities between members of the same sex, is common in adolescents, especially in closed communities such as public schools and service camps. It usually represents a transitory phase and disappears with maturity. Again guilt feelings and emotional distress are common.

Emotional identifications ('crushes', hero-worship and calf-love, etc.) are common, especially in girls. These frustrated, intense, but short-lived identifications with older people — film stars, teachers, etc. — may be a source of distress to the adolescent.

Impotence

In males there are three types of potency disorder: impotence, failure to ejaculate, and premature ejaculation. *Acute onset impotence* occurs in young males, is associated with anxiety, and usually has a definite physical or psychological precipitant. These men usually seek help spontaneously. They do not lose the capacity to respond erotically, retain morning erections, and can masturbate. *Insidious onset impotence* usually begins over the age of 30. There is a gradual onset with no clear precipitant. The man seeks help only at his wife's request. There is a general loss of libido and erotic response. Anxiety is secondary, most often provoked by the complaints of the spouse. Ejaculatory failure may be an early symptom in this group. *Premature ejaculation* is a separate syndrome, not associated with impotence. It has usually been present since puberty, and is found in tense anxious individuals.

Treatment

The acute onset cases respond well to sexual education (usually involving both partners), relaxation therapy and psychotherapy. The more commonly seen insidious onset cases show improvement in only one-third, probably because they are not psychogenic in origin. Aphrodisiacs and hormones are no more effective than placebos.

Frigidity

Frigidity covers a variety of disorders in the female, ranging from lack of interest in coitus and failure to experience orgasm to active distaste, with dyspareunia and vaginismus (involuntary muscular spasm preventing penetration). As in the male there is wide individual variation in female sexual response. Not all women invariably experience orgasm yet many now expect to do so and seek advice if they do not. The menstrual cycle, childbirth and age all have effects on libido. Psychogenic causes of frigidity are much more common than physical or anatomical problems but the latter must be excluded. In severe cases with dyspareunia ('virgin wives') a disturbed relationship with the father is usual, and the woman usually has an hysterical personality.

Motivation is important in determining outcome. If the patient seeks help quickly and of her own volition, rather than after pressure from her husband, response to psychotherapy, often combined with relaxation exercises and the use of graduated dilators, is frequently satisfactory. Sexual counselling of both partners is more helpful than attempts to treat the individual.

Sexual anomalies

Homosexuality, exhibitionism, transvestism, fetishism and sado-masochism fall under this heading. In each case the dividing line between normality and abnormality may be hard to draw; the division is partly social and varies in different cultures.

Homosexuality

Homosexuality is the most frequent anomaly. It is common in adolescence and in all-male communities. It is found in many immature mammals and in all human cultures, in some of which such behaviour evokes no social disapproval. Probably a third of the male population have had some homosexual experience at some time in their lives but only about 4 per cent are exclusively homosexual.

Genetic factors may be of aetiological importance in some cases but there are no endocrine abnormalities and nuclear sex is normal. Contrary to popular belief, the homosexual is rarely abnormal in appearance or manner. In a group of biological intersexes homosexuality has been found to be no more frequent than in the general population. In many cases psychogenic factors predominate, e.g. disturbed parent-child relationship, seductions and traumatic experiences in childhood. The latter accounts for the severe attitude of society to those found guilty of offences against young persons.

The other deviations are less frequent. In general, psychological factors predominate in the aetiology but any person first presenting in later life with complaints in this field may be suffering from associated physical disease, e.g. enlarged prostate, early dementia.

Treatment. Many deviants never seek treatment or are seen by the psychiatrist only when legal offences have been committed. Such cases, without adequate motivation for treatment, can rarely be helped. Some patients present with symptoms (anxiety, depression) which mask or obscure the fundamental difficulties. Others (usually young adults) may seek help directly in the solution of their psychosexual difficulties.

Each case must be considered in the light of the circumstances of the referral, the history, the patient's attitude to his anomaly and the nature and severity of any associated psychiatric condition.

Stilboestrol in large doses may be used to suppress libido temporarily. Psychotherapy, in suitable cases, may deal with the psychosexual problems, or help the patient to live with his anomaly without clashing with society. Aversion by behaviour therapy techniques may be useful in selected cases. Complete cure is infrequent.

Termination of pregnancy

Since the Abortion Act, 1968 (see p. 100) large numbers of pregnancies have been terminated on 'mental health' grounds.

Doctors vary widely in their interpretation of the social and psychiatric spirit of the Act, but there has been an increasing tendency, in face of changing public opinion, to provide abortion on demand. It can be argued that there are few or no psychiatric grounds for termination — the severely mental subnormal and the chronically schizophrenic do not suffer a deterioration in health through pregnancy, and the fact that they would be unable to care for the child is not legal ground for termination. Conversely it has been argued by other psychiatrists that continuing an unwanted pregnancy will always have adverse effects on the mental health of the mother.

Extensive follow-up studies since the Act show that very few women who have had terminations experience severe remorse or depression as a result, regardless of religious affiliation. Equally, in those refused, no serious mental illness occurs, although unhappiness and social distress may result and the unwanted children may suffer subsequently.

Puerperal illnesses

Psychosis

Prevalence — 1 in 1000 births. Not an entity and classified as affective, schizophrenic, etc., rather than 'puerperal psychosis'. Patient usually well for first few days post-partum; 60 per cent begin in first month, 80 per cent within three months. Only 1 per cent organic, remainder affective or schizophrenic. Often atypical symptoms in first week, with some clouding of consciousness. Differential diagnosis: puerperal cerebral thrombo-phlebitis, distinguished by neurological signs. Treatment and prognosis as for other affective and schizophrenic illnesses. Risk of recurrence in future pregnancies is one in five, i.e. more than 100 times the post-partum risk in general population.

Neurosis

Most mothers experience transient weepiness and poor concentration in the week after delivery (post-partum blues). Neurotic depression is common in the first year, usually after the first child in young, anxious women, often of below average intelligence and over-dependent on their own mothers. They show anxiety, depression and have difficulty in coping with the baby.

Most psychiatric units provide facilities for admitting mothers and babies, and find them helpful in treating both psychoses and neuroses in the puerperium.

FURTHER READING

Berne, E. *Sex in Human Loving*. Penguin.
Comfort, A. *Sex in Society*. Penguin.
Schofield, M. *The Sexual Behaviour of Young People*. Penguin.
Storr, A. *Sexual Deviation*. Penguin.

14. Psychiatry and Physical Illness

The psychosomatic approach

There are two main approaches. One is 'holistic', believing that in any physical illness psychological and social factors must be considered for a full understanding of the patient and the illness; naturally they will be more relevant in some patients than in others. The second view is more limited, restricting the term to diseases in which stress or emotion may produce physical changes in organs supplied by the autonomic nervous system, and asserting that certain types of personality are associated with certain disorders.

Clinical applications

There are several diseases in which personality factors seem to be associated with the disease, in which stress precedes the onset, and whose course varies with the patient's life situation. Migraine, peptic ulcer, irritable bowel syndrome, asthma and eczema are generally accepted examples. The patient with *migraine* tends to be intelligent, conscientious and to show obsessional personality traits. Migraine attacks are often related to periods of stress or repressed hostility, but typically the attack occurs only when the situation has passed and the stress is over — 'weekend migraine'.

Much early work on the 'psychosomatic personality' is unsound but recent research on *hypertension* shows such patients to be emotionally labile, easily upset, and scoring midway between a normal and a neurotic group on tests of neuroticism. There is also convincing research relating coronary artery disease to life styles. Such connections are complex and many aetiological factors are involved. If a full psychiatric history is taken in patients with physical illness social and personality factors will be revealed which may often assist in clinical management and treatment.

Psychophysiological aspects

Hypothalamic lesions in animals produce gastro-intestinal disorders. The neurophysiological and neuroendocrine pathways by which acute stress affects the body are now well established. Behavioural stress applied to animals, either by restraining them or by shock avoidance (Brady's 'executive monkeys'), also produces gastric ulceration and other gastrointestinal disorders. More recently it has been shown that autonomic responses, e.g. heart rate, can be altered by operant conditioning. It may be that faulty instrumental conditioning plays a part in producing psychosomatic disorder, and conditioning and the use of bio-feedback techniques may soon play a part in treatment. It is difficult to apply the results of acute stress experiments to the situations of chronic stress which are thought to determine human psychosomatic disorders.

Life events and illness

The effects of severe sustained stress have been studied in the survivors of concentration camps and prisoners of war. Such groups, apart from psychiatric sequelae, show an increase in dyspepsia and peptic ulceration, and have a higher mortality from many causes.

There is evidence from the study of life events in relation to illness that significant clusters of illnesses may occur in individuals after periods of increased stress.

Of the normal life stresses to which the individual is exposed, *bereavement* is usually rated the most severe and will frequently lead to the patient seeking medical help.

Acute grief typically lasts for 6 to 12 weeks, but significant disturbance persists for one to two years. The first phase, lasting up to two weeks after the death, is of protective numbness, with dissociation and depersonalisation. The bereaved person in this state may cope very adequately with funeral arrangements and outwardly appear surprisingly unmoved, or 'shocked'. This is succeeded by intense grief and distress, with restlessness, attacks of sighing and choking sensations. Over the first three months this gradually gives way to constant depression of variable degree. There is difficulty in communicating, vivid dreams of the dead person, and illusions of the dead person's presence are common.

Recognition of this reaction is important for several reasons:

1. Death tends increasingly to be a *taboo topic,* to the extent that bereaved people are stigmatised. Little allowance is made for the normal process of mourning to take place.

2. It must be distinguished from *atypical grief,* where the reaction is not only unduly severe or prolonged, but is often characterised by excessive guilt and self-blame, hypo-chondriasis, and suicidal ideas.

3. The period of bereavement carries a high morbidity and mortality, not only from suicide. Comparison with control groups shows that in the year after a death the bereaved (particularly widowers) consult their doctors more often, are prescribed more drugs, have higher suicide rates and have higher death rates from other causes.

FURTHER READING

Munro, A. *Psychosomatic Medicine.* Penguin.

15. Psychiatric Problems of Old Age

As with other branches of medicine the number of elderly patients referred to psychiatric services has risen steeply in recent years. In some parts of the country, e.g. retirement areas in the South of England, the proportion of people over 65 years in the population has reached 30 per cent. In most districts the figure is at least 12 per cent. Mental changes are a part of normal aging. All old people decline in intellectual power, show narrowing of interest and outlook, are unable to accept new ideas and tend to dwell on the past. Mental illness in old age shows such changes in an exaggerated form.

Although elderly people suffer from a wide range of mental illnesses the major problem is that of *senile dementia* and *arteriosclerotic dementia* (see p. 31). The incidence of dementing illness rises with increasing age and about 30 per cent of individuals over the age of 75 years suffer from some degree of dementia. Clearly not every dementing patient can be given hospital admission and there is increasing interest in the organisation of out-patient and community services to help them and their relatives. Elderly people with mental disorder should, ideally, be medically assessed by a psychiatrist and a geriatrician working together. In some areas a joint psychiatric/geriatric assessment unit has been established.

Where the main problem is that of disturbed behaviour, e.g. wandering, aggressiveness, paranoid delusions, then long term care in a psychiatric hospital may be necessary. Where no special behaviour disorder exists the patient should, if possible, be cared for in a *residential home* provided by the local authority. If there is a significant degree of physical illness as well as mental disorder, long term geriatric care will be required. Many mildly demented elderly people can remain at home provided there is adequate domiciliary support. This can take the form of a home help, home meals service, chiropody, physiotherapy, etc. The *health visitor* plays a major part in supervising the home care of the elderly. *Voluntary services* also play an increasing part in this branch of psychiatry.

Elderly people also frequently suffer from *affective illness*. This will usually respond to the treatment prescribed for affective illness in younger people. However affective illness in the elderly is frequently associated with co-existing physical illness and every effort should be made to restore the patient to optimum physical health. Deafness may precipitate affective and *paranoid illness* in the elderly. Bereavement is a common experience for elderly people and the loss of a spouse, particularly of a wife, is frequently followed by a depressive illness in which social isolation, self neglect, poor nutrition, etc., may eventually lead to the development of a confusional state and admission to a geriatric or psychiatric unit. *Psychoneurosis* is less often diagnosed in older patients but does occur. States of anxiety and reactive depression related to retirement, bereavement, financial difficulty, social isolation and fear of failing physical abilities will require psychological treatment (see Chap. 21).

FURTHER READING

Bromley, D. B. *The Psychology of Human Ageing*. Penguin.
Townsend, P. *The Family Life of Old People*. Penguin.

16. Suicide

Suicide and parasuicide — the more recent and neutral term for attempted suicide — are major topics in current psychiatry, because of the increasing numbers involved and the research they have produced. In the world over 1000 suicides take place daily; in Britain there are over 3000 deaths from suicide annually, and parasuicide is 10 times as common. Self-poisoning now accounts for 15 per cent of all medical admissions, and in patients under 40 years is the commonest cause of admission to hospital medical units.

Suicide is an emotional subject. Several myths are in common circulation: that suicide happens without warning; that those who threaten suicide never do so; that all attempted suicides are attention-seeking and trivial; and that all suicides are mentally ill. All are false. Suicides and parasuicides are two overlapping populations. Suicides tend to be over 45, male, of higher social class and use violent methods; parasuicides tend to be under 45, female, of lower social class, and use self-poisoning.

Parasuicide

The *diagnosis* in the majority of cases is depression, more often neurotic than endogenous. Many have personality disorders, either immature, or aggressive and antisocial. Many are alcoholics or drug addicts — in a Glasgow study 70 per cent of all self-poisoners had been drinking at the time of the attempt. Few schizophrenics make attempts. In some cases no formal diagnosis can be made; there is usually a history of an impulsive reaction to acute social distress.

Motives are mixed. Apart from the wish to die, many are seeking aid (the 'Cry for Help'), some are punishing or manipulating family or friends, and some are appealing to fate by gambling with their lives. The *methods* used are increasingly dominated by drugs, particularly barbiturates, aspirin and psychotropic drugs.

Prognosis. After an attempt, 1 in 50 will go on to kill themselves within a year, and in the 10 year period after attempts about 10 per cent will kill themselves and 25 per cent repeat the attempt.

Suicide

Much is known about the general characteristics of groups of suicides. They are predominantly male, old and single, divorced or widowed. They are socially isolated, or have lost status through loss of employment or retirement. Suicide is more common in social classes 1 and 2 and in certain occupations (doctors, dentists and university students). There may be a history of physical illness, commonly painful and chronic, of recent bereavement, or of alcoholism or drug abuse. High rates are linked with high density of population and residence in cities. Frequently there is a history of a broken home in childhood.

Clinically, two main groups of successful suicides can be distinguished. The first have no history of a previous attempt, have stable if dependent previous personalities, and kill themselves without warning, using drastic methods (e.g. hanging, drowning). Often their death is precipitated by bereavement, usually the loss of a spouse. The second have a history of a previous parasuicide. They are often severely disordered personalities, with long histories of poor work records, psychiatric treatment, heavy drinking or criminality. They die from self-poisoning, after warning others, and often with others in the vicinity.

Management and prevention

Apart from medical management of the parasuicide, any attempt, however trivial or impulsive it may appear, merits careful psychiatric history-taking and examination. The past history, the precipitants and setting of the attempt, and the history and attitudes of immediate relatives are worth special attention. The mood of the patient in the first 48 hours may be deceptively cheerful, but few mistakes will be made if an adequate history is taken.

Prevention on a large scale must be directed to measures to counter or minimise social isolation. The Samaritans and other suicide agencies have had some success with depressed potential suicides. The early diagnosis and treatment of psychiatric disorder, with ready admission to hospital of patients showing the high risk factors discussed, is important. All doctors have a duty to restrict access to drugs by avoiding large or repeated prescriptions. The increasing change to natural gas is also helpful — asphyxia is less lethal than carbon monoxide poisoning.

FURTHER READING

Alvarez, A. *The Savage God*. Penguin.
Stengel, E. *Suicide and Attempted Suicide*. Penguin.

17. Mental Handicap

Mental handicap (amentia, oligophrenia) is a defect of intelligence existing from birth or from an early age. The English Mental Health Act, 1959, prefers 'mental subnormality' and recognises subnormality and severe subnormality. The Scottish Act of 1960 retains the older 'mental deficiency' and makes no subdivision. While low intelligence is essential, a low IQ is not the sole criterion. Personality and associated physical defects have significant effects on educability, and social competence has always been the main diagnostic criterion.

Prevalence

Two to three per cent of the population have some degree of mental handicap; they are gradually identified between birth and 14 years, after which the figure remains steady. Some 70 per cent live in the community. For every case of severe subnormality (IQ less than 30) there are 4 cases of moderate subnormality (IQ less than 50) and 15 mild cases of mild subnormality (IQ less than 75). Severe cases have a prevalence of $3 \cdot 7/1000$. Subnormality is nine times more common in social class 5 than in social class 1 and 2. It is higher in rural areas, and in males ($1 \cdot 3$ to 1). There is a family history of subnormality in 17 per cent and of mental illness in 4 per cent.

Aetiology

There are two main types — organic and subcultural. The latter group comprises those individuals of low intelligence who can be expected to occur at one tail of the normal distribution curve. Intelligence is normally distributed in the population, and most intelligence tests are standardised with a mean IQ of 100 and a standard deviation of 15. The subnormal population is usually defined as having an IQ of more than two standard deviations below the mean, i.e. an IQ under 70. The rates quoted above for different degrees of defect illustrate the effects of the probability distribution and sub-cultural defect. In severe defect — below IQ 50 — there are higher numbers than would be expected by chance (a 'bulge in the tail'), and the vast majority of this group have organic brain disease, compared with only 25 to 50 per cent in those with IQ's of 50 to 70.

Multiple handicap is common. A substantial minority have associated psychosis or neurosis, and up to 40 per cent show difficult behaviour in childhood. Accompanying handicaps include poor physical development, sensory defects such as deafness and poor vision, cerebral palsy and epilepsy. Few with severe handicap can find employment, but above IQ 50 education, upbringing, social class and temperament, together with associated handicaps all play a part in the final achievement or failure.

Diagnosis and assessment

Antenatal

Amniocentesis: a developing area of early diagnosis. Tissue culture used to detect chromosomal abnormalities, enzyme defects and sex of the infant. May prove useful in older mothers with high risk of Down's syndrome, if an existing child has a genetic defect and risk is high, or if the disorder suspected is sex linked. Alphafoetoprotein estimation in amniotic fluid and blood now used to detect neural tube defects (spina-bifida).

Infancy

Always suspect subnormality when there has been anoxia and when there is low birth weight, dysplasia, cerebral palsy, convulsions or small cranial circumference. Probably 1 per cent of live births show serious retardation, but at 7 years only 0.4 per cent have IQ's below 50, the effect of *selective mortality*.

Investigations in suspected cases include chromosome studies, amino-acid chromatography, specific blood and urine tests for inborn errors of metabolism and detection of specific antibodies in mother and child. Developmental scales are available for diagnosis in infancy and childhood.

Childhood: many identified by failure to stand, walk or talk at the normal times.

School: milder degrees of subnormality are commonly diagnosed in the early school years through educational difficulties.

Classification

Organic causes
1. Prior to conception
   a. Chromosomal, e.g. Down's syndrome
   b. Genetic, single, e.g. inborn errors, or multifactorial
2. Pre-natal and peri-natal
   a. Maternal infections (rubella, toxoplasmosis, syphilis, cytomegalic inclusion body disease)
   b. Fetal infections (encephalopathies, maternal toxaemia)
   c. Maternal malnutrition — rare
   d. Perinatal damage (hypoxia, birth injury)
   e. Kernicterus.

Down's syndrome (mongolism)

Described by John Langdon Down in 1866. Due to chromosomal abnormality. Various forms, but 90 per cent due to trisomy 21, an extra small acrocentric chromosome in group G, giving 47 rather than 46 chromosomes. Caused by nondisjunction during meiosis of the oöcyte, i.e. the ovum is involved and not the sperm. More common in older mothers; compared with a 25-year-old mother, a mother of 40 has 20 times the risk and a mother aged 45, 50 times the risk. Mongols born to young mothers usually show a different abnormality: translocation, in which there are 46 chromosomes, one of which is large and atypical. Clinically, mongolism is common: 1 in 700 live births, but up to 50 per cent die in the first year. Mongols formerly had a short life due to infection, but those who survive infancy now live longer. All show varying degrees of subnormality. In infancy hypotonia and hyperflexibility are found. There are multiple abnormalities: microcephaly, flat face, sloping eyes with epicanthic fold, big tongue and short neck; broad, flat hands with Simian crease and short fingers; congenital heart lesions, infertility, temperament jovial, often musical. In early pregnancy may now be identified by amniotic cell culture.

Metabolic abnormalities

Acquired
   a. Hypoglycaemia
   b. Hyperbilirubinaemia (Kernicterus)
   c. Hypothyroidism (Cretinism)
   d. Hypoproteinaemia
   e. Hypercalcaemia
   f. Lead poisoning

Inborn
   a. Lipid
   b. Carbohydrate
   c. Amino acids.

Inborn errors of metabolism are interesting but very rare: acquired abnormalities are four times as common.

Acquired metabolic abnormality

Kernicterus: from Rh or ABO incompatibility or in prematurity. When level of unconjugated serum bilirubin exceeds 20 mg/100 ml, damage takes place in basal ganglia and cerebellum. Often hypertonus, cyanosis, convulsions with later choreo-athetosis, deafness and subnormality. Antenatal detection and exchange transfusion.

Hypothyroidism (Cretinism) has various causes: enzyme deficiencies, absent or maldeveloped thyroid, ingestion of drugs, e.g. phenylbutazone, PAS. Symptoms include: persistent jaundice, lethargy, protruding tongue and umbilical hernia; early thyroid treatment essential.

Inborn metabolic abnormality

All autosomal recessives. Rare — 1 in 10 000 to 1 in 50 000. Caused by deficient enzyme blocking a metabolic reaction: symptoms arise from accumulation of lipids, carbohydrate or amino acids before the block, or deficiency beyond the block.

Lipid disorders include Tay-Sachs' disease (ganglioside), Gaucher's disease (cerebroside) and Niemann-Pick disease (sphingomyelin). Commoner in Jews, begin early, have a rapid fatal course.

Connective tissue disorders (mucopoly-saccharoidoses) include Hurler's syndrome (gargoylism).

Carbohydrate disorders include galactosaemia, in which there is jaundice, cataracts, proteinuria and galactosuria. Treatable.

Amino acid disorders: best known is phenylketonuria. Infants are screened by Guthrie inhibition test on blood for raised phenylalanine levels. The defect is in transforming phenylalanine to tyrosine from a deficiency of the enzyme phenylalanine hydroxylase. Occurs 1 in 12 000 births. No physical abnormalities, but often have blue eyes, fair hair and dermatitis. Treatment: phenylalanine free diet — variable results.

Neurological defects

Sturge-Weber syndrome: naevoid defect. Fits, hemiplegia, naevi (port wine stains) especially on face and neck. Venous angioma of pia; calcification of skull on X-ray. Hemispherectomy may help.

Tuberous sclerosis (epiloia). Sclerotic nodules in brain, epilepsy. Tumours elsewhere, especially kidneys and heart. Epilepsy. Skin lesions: adenoma sebaceum, fibromatosis, phakomata.

Laurence-Moon-Biedl Syndrome: mental defect, pigmentary degeneration of the retinae, obesity, hypogenitalism, polydactyly. Usually familial.

Bony defects

Genetic microcephaly: probably single recessive gene.

Hypertelorism: great breadth between eyes, due to abnormality of base of skull.

Oxycephaly: tower skull or steeple-head. Rarely associated with defect. Hypertelorism and oxycephaly need not be associated with subnormality.

Treatment and care

Patients should be cared for at home where possible but the stresses on other members of the family must be weighed. Boredom and overcrowding produce disturbed behaviour, and drugs (e.g. anticonvulsants) may further impair performance. Education is essential and should emphasise practical social skills — learning to wash, dress, eat, travel and work. Subnormals with an IQ of 50 or over can benefit from some form of schooling. Most defectives in the community are capable of some form of work and this may be in an occupation centre or sheltered workshop if open employment cannot be found. Very severely handicapped cases, cases with multiple handicaps or complicated by severe behaviour disorder (e.g. aggressiveness, disinhibited sexual behaviour) or psychotic illnesses will require care in hospital possibly throughout life. Prevention involves the paediatrician and obstetrician. Genetic counselling is developing in importance.

18. Child and Adolescent Psychiatry

Classification

A World Health Organisation Committee recommended that children be assessed on four dimensions: (1) clinical psychiatric syndrome; (2) intelligence; (3) organic factors and (4) psychosocial factors. Clinically, children show the same range of psychiatric disorders as adults: psychoneurosis, psychosomatic disorders and psychosis. The vast majority can be divided into two groups:

1. With predominantly neurotic symptoms. These children suffer from anxiety, phobias, shyness, sleep and appetite disorders and tics. Most grow up to be stable adults.

2. With predominantly conduct disorders: stealing, aggression, lying, over-activity, truancy. Poor prognosis in adult life with much crime, alcoholism, psychiatric admission, poor work record.

Children with behaviour disorders are usually disturbed either at home or at school; only in severe cases at both. About 7 per cent of 10 to 11 year olds have some kind of psychiatric disorder. Boys have twice as much as girls and more often have conduct disorders.

A few disorders are specific to childhood and adolescence, e.g. early childhood *autism,* the *hyperkinetic syndrome* and *anorexia nervosa. Specific developmental disorders* include dyslexia, stammering, enuresis, encopresis and 'clumsy children'.

Specific syndromes

Nocturnal enuresis

Common in early years. At 14 years drops to 1 in 35. More frequent in males of below average intelligence living in poor social conditions. Strong family history. Five per cent urinary infections. May be neurotic, e.g. regression after birth of a younger sibling, or developmental. Treatment: conditioning by pad and bell (see p. 106), Imipramine 25 or 50mg at night in older children; prolonged treatment is necessary. *Encopresis:* Soiling; rarer than enuresis. Usually retention with overflow. Normal intelligence; may be neurotic or developmental. Treatment: unrewarding, but 50 per cent spontaneous recovery in two years, and all recover before adult life.

Stuttering

Two groups. First are dull, poor social background, often birth injury. The second, average or above average intelligence, ambitious families with worrying obsessional mothers. In both groups the anxiety engendered by stuttering may lead to secondary neurotic disorders. Speech therapy helpful.

Early childhood autism

A form of childhood psychosis beginning from birth or in the first three years. Not schizophrenia, which is rare and occurs later in childhood. Now generally agreed to be an organic condition — formerly attributed to unbringing or the parents' personalities. The central defect is a difficulty in comprehension and the use of language. Rare — about 1 in 2000 school children. Three boys affected for every girl. Parents tend to be intelligent. Symptoms comprise lack of speech comprehension, mutism or abnormal speech, with echolalia, avoidance of the personal pronoun, monotonous mechanical voice. Difficulty in copying movements, flicking movements of hands, spinning and jumping movements. Paradoxical response to sounds. Resistance to change of routine. Socially aloof, live in a world of their own. Often tantrums. When testable, only 30 per cent have an IQ above 55. A third develop fits in adolescence or adult life. Differential diagnosis: deafness, partial blindness, elective mutism, mental subnormality. Prognosis: poor. Sixty per cent unchanged, only 15 per cent find open employment. Best with higher IQs.

School refusal ('School phobia')

Relatively rare. Peak age 11 to 12 years. Often precipitated by change of school or illness in parents, grandparents. Mostly boys, intelligence average. Well behaved children doing well at school, often anxious and shy. Increasing anxiety, often with abdominal pain and vomiting, culminating in refusal to go to school. Quite distinct from truancy. Mothers often over-protective, subject to depression. Most due to separation anxiety rather than fear of school. Treatment may necessitate admission, residential school or temporary separation from parents.

Hyperkinetic syndrome

Associated with minimal brain damage. Onset 3 to 4 years. Restless impulsive and distractable children whose learning is impaired by poor attention. Paradoxical response to drugs: helped by amphetamines and Ritalin and made worse by barbiturates. Chlorpromazine also used.

Elective mutism

Neurotic disorder in which child, usually male, is persistently mute in selected circumstances, e.g. at school. Most are solitary, over-dependent on parents. Treatment by change of environment or admission.

Anorexia nervosa

Common and increasing disorder of adolescent girls. Occurs in 1 in 150 girls in this age group. Only 1 in 20 patients are male. Begins with wish to diet and feeling fat. Progressive weight loss with early amenorrhoea, patient quickly becomes emaciated, but maintains she feels normal and looks normal. Claims to be eating adequately. Often self-induced vomiting and excessive purging: both in secret. May be intermittent over-eating (bulimia) especially after treatment. Patient very resistant to accepting treatment. Potentially serious. In those whom the condition lasts for ten years the later mortality may be 10 per cent.

Weight falls in typical case to 30 to 35 kg. Best regarded as a phobic avoidance of adolescent weight gain and the physical and psychological changes of puberty. Treatment: target weight of at least 50 kg must be set and agreed. In-patient care usually essential with good nursing, high doses of phenothiazines and psychotherapy. Extended and careful follow-up.

Treatment methods

In emotional disorders family relationships may be relevant and most child psychiatric clinics employ a treatment team including doctor, social worker, psychologist, nurse and play therapist. Individual or group therapy with the family members as well as the child are used. Residential treatment in hospital or special boarding school may be needed when the home is unsatisfactory or where the behaviour disorder cannot be contained by out-patient care alone. Drug treatments are less often used than with adults but tranquillisers and antidepressants are of value. ECT and psychosurgery are seldom, if ever, needed.

FURTHER READING

Barker, P. *Basic Child Psychiatry*. Staples.
Stone, F. H. & Koupernik, C. *Child Psychiatry for Students*. Churchill Livingstone.
Valentine, C. W. *The Normal Child and Some of his Abnormalities*. Penguin.
Winnicott, D. W. *The Child, the Family and the Outside World*. Penguin.

19. Forensic Psychiatry

More than other doctors, the psychiatrist comes into contact with the law. Psychiatric patients, because of their disturbed behaviour, are likely to clash with society — hence the Mental Health Acts — and may encounter the police or the courts as a result. Forensic psychiatry is a growing subject, because there is growing interest in research, prevention, treatment and rehabilitation of the criminal rather than simple punishment. Not all criminals, of course, suffer from a psychiatric abnormality; one of the doctor's tasks is to distinguish those who do. This chapter gives a brief selection of psychiatrically important topics.

Crime

Crime is associated with youth and the male sex. There are 9 male offenders for every female and 33 male prisoners for every female. The largest increases in crime in the last 30 years have been in males between 14 and 21 years and the highest rates for theft and violent offences are in this age group. Studies of young male offenders show that they are of mesomorphic body build, extraverted, emotionally unstable, and condition poorly — they do not learn quickly from experience or punishment. They come from large families where there has been little parental control or from broken homes, are usually intellectually dull, of lower social class, and from areas of high crime.

Publicity gives a false impression of sex offences and crimes of violence which account for less than 5 per cent of all offences. About 2 per cent of all offenders are psychotic or mentally defective. Special hospitals for psychiatric patients who are potentially dangerous or criminal account for less than 1 per cent of psychiatric beds. There are more epileptics in the prison population than would be expected, but they are no more likely to commit violent crimes.

Violent criminals are of two types: under-controlled, habitually aggressive men with records of repeated minor violence (65 per cent have abnormal EEG's); over-controlled, older men who commit a single act of major violence, usually involving a relative (24 per cent have abnormal EEG's).

Murder is rare. It is associated with drinking (55 per cent in a Scottish series) and with subsequent suicide of the murderer (10 per cent in Scotland, up to 30 per cent in England). Matricide is very rare but is associated with schizophrenia. Two syndromes can be identified as a major risk: (a) the *sadistic murderer* with interests in black magic, Nazi souvenirs, guns and bondage perversions; and (b) *morbid jealousy* (Othello syndrome) which accounts for 10 per cent of murders — the man developes a delusional belief in the infidelity of his wife and there is a 5 year history of a well developed paranoid delusional system, with complicated searches for non-existent evidence.

XYY syndrome

At the State Hospital Carstairs in 1965, 9 of 315 male patients were found to have abnormal sex chromosome complements, in the form of an extra Y chromosome — the XYY karyotype. The finding was confirmed in other institutions for psychiatric offenders, and shown to be associated with height (average 5 ft 10 in), below average intelligence, and a record of crime against property from an early age. The patients did not usually come from criminal families or cultures. The percentage is higher than in the general population but it is estimated that for every XYY identified there must be 100 'at large', and the significance of the findings remains uncertain.

Shoplifting

The main female crime. Only 6 per cent are professionals, 60 per cent are foreign born. Many are teenagers but there is a large group in the 45 to 55 age group. In first offenders 20 per cent have psychiatric symptoms, in recidivists 30 per cent. One third have gynaecological symptoms, some menopausal but usually pre or post-natal or post-hysterectomy. In a 10 year follow-up 9 per cent required in-patient psychiatric treatment. The psychiatric symptoms are depressive. There is usually evidence of repressed resentment and ideas of self-punishment. In these cases the shop-lifting is impulsive with little or no attempt at concealment. It is often provoked by a depressing event, but the woman frequently denies problems which are obvious to others.

Prostitution

Prostitutes have a high incidence of mental abnormality. A study of a prison population showed that 25 per cent were alcoholic, 25 per cent were drug dependent, 25 per cent had a history of parasuicide, and 25 per cent had a variety of physical deformities and illnesses. Fifteen per cent were, or had been, psychiatrically ill, and 15 per cent were homosexual or bisexual.

Battered babies

There are four main types of child damage: *Infanticide,* in which a mentally ill or defective mother kills her infant; *the wasted and neglected child,* the product of an inadequate mother and home; *deliberate sustained cruelty* by a sadistic parent; and *the battered baby syndrome,* increasingly reported in recent years.

The *child* is usually 3 years, there is a delay in reporting injury, denial of assault and a discrepancy between history and findings. There may be bruising, subdural haematoma, single or multiple fractures, ruptured liver and typical lacerations inside the mouth. Usually one particular child in the family is singled out, often the first or the last. One-third are illegitimate or unwanted. The *parents* are in their twenties, the mother of low intelligence, pregnant or premenstrual, the father unemployed and with a criminal record. The parents were sometimes ill-treated in their own childhood. They are superficially co-operative, the child is well dressed and well nourished, but there are marital and financial problems. Few are psychopathic or mentally ill.

Thorough investigation is necessary in suspected cases. The family doctor may not suspect the possibility of battering. The future safety of the children is paramount. If no-one intervenes there is a 60 per cent chance of further injury or death, and a 1 in 13 chance of a subsequent child being battered. Many agencies must be involved in care and follow-up on a team basis.

FURTHER READING

Patrick, J. *A Glasgow Gang Observed*. Methuen.

20. Legal Aspects of Psychiatry

In contrast with other forms of illness, admission of all psychiatric patients to mental hospitals was in the past governed by legal procedures laid down in the *Lunacy and Mental Deficiency Acts.*

The latest Mental Health Acts (England 1959, Scotland 1960) provide for the care and treatment of mentally disordered persons, for their protection and for safeguarding their property and affairs. They ensure that wherever possible the mentally disordered patient can have the same ready access, without formality, to care and treatment as the patient suffering from a physical disorder.

The Mental Health (Scotland) Act, 1960

Mental disorder is used as a general term to cover *mental illness* and *mental deficiency,* however manifested or caused. These are the only categories of mental disorder referred to in the Act.

Particular hospitals are no longer designated as mental hospitals or mental deficiency institutions. Special provision is made for 'State Hospitals' for patients with dangerous, violent or criminal propensities who require treatment under conditions of special security.

Provision of mental health services by local authorities

Local authorities are empowered to:

1. Provide residential accommodation
2. Exercise functions in respect of persons under guardianship, and supervise mental defectives
3. Ascertain mental deficiency in persons not of school age
4. Appoint Mental Health Officers (M.H.O.) to carry out duties relating to compulsory detention and guardianship
5. Provide ancillary and supplementary services.

The local authority must also arrange suitable training for mental defectives not already provided for by special schools.

Admission to hospital

It is specifically stated that nothing in the Act is to prevent a patient requiring treatment for mental disorder from being admitted to any hospital or nursing home and receiving treatment without formality, in the same way as patients are admitted to hospital for treatment for physical conditions.

Compulsory admission.

(Section 24). Where the patient is unwilling to enter hospital the Act provides for:

1. Admission on the application of the nearest relative or a M.H.O., the recommendation of two doctors, and the approval of a Sheriff prior to admission

2. Subsequent periodic review of the need for detention

3. Right of appeal to the Sheriff against detention by patient or nearest relative

4. An independent central authority, the Mental Welfare Commission, with a right to visit patients, discharge a patient at any time and to hear and investigate any complaint of wrongful or improper treatment.

The two medical practitioners must examine the patient separately. One must have special experience in the diagnosis or treatment of mental disorder and the other, where possible, should be the patient's general practitioner. Only one of the doctors may be on the staff of the hospital to which the patient is to be admitted and neither if the patient is to be treated privately.

The medical recommendations state:

1. The form of the patient's mental disorder (i.e. mental illness or mental deficiency)

2. That it is of a nature or degree warranting detention in hospital for treatment

3. That the interests of the patient's health and safety or the protection of other persons cannot otherwise be secured.

The Sheriff must approve the applications and medical recommendations and may make his own enquiries. If the nearest relative objects he must be given a hearing in private. The completed Section 24 Order then permits detention in hospital for 28 days.

Emergency admission (Section 31). A patient may be

removed to hospital on the strength of one medical recommendation in cases of urgency and detained for up to seven days. The recommendation must state that mental illness exists and where possible that consent of a relative has been obtained. The hospital which agrees to accept the patient usually arranges transport and escorts. During the seven day period the Section 24 Order should be completed.

Two classes of patient are not liable to compulsory admission if over 21:

1. Mental defectives who are able to lead an independent life and guard themselves against serious exploitation

2. Mentally ill persons with a persistent disorder manifested only by abnormally aggressive or seriously irresponsible conduct.

Patients in these classes already detained are to be reviewed with a view to discharge on reaching the age of 25.

Part V of the Act deals with patients concerned in criminal proceedings. Courts may remand offenders to hospital for a psychiatric report (Section 54). After trial the Court may make an Order for treatment (Section 55). In certain circumstances a restriction may be placed on a patient's discharge from hospital. (Section 60). A patient who is 'insane and unfit to plead' with automatically be dealt with under Section 63 and receive a treatment order.

The Mental Welfare Commission is a statutory body set up by the Scottish Act to exercise a protective function for persons with mental disorder: it can investigate complaints by patients or their relatives about their treatment.

The Mental Health Act 1959 (England)

There are some important differences in detail between the Scottish and English Mental Health Acts. For example, in Scotland the Acts refer to Mental Illness and Mental Deficiency. In the English Acts the terms used are Mental Illness, Subnormality (and Severe Subnormality) and Psychopathic Disorder.

In England no judicial approval is needed for compulsory admission and the functions of the Scottish Mental Welfare Commission are carried out by regional Mental Health Review Tribunals.

Legal considerations

Care and treatment of the psychiatric patient may involve a number of other legal considerations. For example:

Marriage and divorce

Husband or wife can obtain divorce on grounds of incurable insanity of the partner. Partner must have been continuously under care and treatment for mental illness for five years.

Marriage can be annulled if one of the parties at the time of the marriage was not able to understand the marriage contract or unable to manage his affairs. The patient, having recovered, can bring an action of nullity. Conversely, a petition for nullity will be upheld if the petitioner was unaware of the partner's insanity at the time of marriage, provided less than one year has elapsed since marriage.

Sterilisation and abortion

In Britain sterilisation and therapeutic termination of pregnancy may be carried out legally for medical reasons; the procedure and indications for termination are now regulated by the Abortion Act, 1967. The grounds recognised by the Act include risk to the life of the pregnant woman, risk of injury to the physical or mental health of the pregnant woman, risk of injury to the physical or mental health of the existing children of the family and substantial risk of physical or mental abnormality or serious handicap in the unborn child. The indications are broad and their interpretation in practice has not yet been established. The abortion is carried out with the permission of the patient on the recommendation of two doctors and has to be notified to the Chief Medical Officer of the Department of Health.

Criminal responsibility

The psychiatric state of the offender is given consideration in all types of legal proceeding. If minor offences occur in a person under psychiatric care he is seldom prosecuted. Attempted suicide is not a legal offence. It is common for an offender to be remanded for a medical report or to be placed on probation on the undertaking that he will accept medical treatment.

In more serious offences the accused may be found insane

and unfit to plead and may be detained in a State Hospital.

Diminished responsibility

Lesser degrees of psychiatric abnormality than insanity are taken into account where mental responsibility is impaired, e.g. by low intelligence or psychopathic personality, and in cases of homicide only, the charge may be reduced from murder to manslaughter by this defence.

Neurotic illness

A diagnosis of psychoneurosis may be considered in mitigation of sentence in minor offences but here legal responsibility is not diminished.

Property of mentally disordered persons

The law provides for the appointment of a *curator bonis* to manage the patient's affairs and the local authority has a duty to arrange for such an appointment if no other person has done so.

21. Psychotherapy

Psychotherapy may be broadly defined as any treatment designed to influence behaviour by verbal or non-verbal means, and includes techniques as varied as confession, reassurance, hypnosis, psychoanalysis and brain-washing. There is ample evidence from outside medicine that what one person says to another may greatly influence behaviour, and doctors have always realised the therapeutic, as well as the diagnostic value of intelligent history-taking. Historically much treatment relied on suggestion, reassurance and the doctor's prestige, administered directly or through placebo therapy. The doctor-patient relationship remains immeasurably important in all specialties.

Such psychotherapy is informal, unplanned, and usually lacks any theoretical foundation. Formal psychotherapy proceeds in a planned way and is based on a theory explaining the psychogenesis of the patient's complaints and the relationship between doctor and patient.

Psychoanalysis

All modern psychotherapy owes much to Sigmund Freud (1856-1939), the originator of the theory and technique of psychoanalysis. Psychoanalysis stresses the role of unconscious forces in neurotic behaviour, easily proven in experimental hypnosis; psychological determinism (the view that phenomena such as dreams and slips of the tongue are not chance occurrences); psychogenesis and the later effects of childhood experiences; and mental mechanisms as defences against anxiety. In technique, Freud developed the use of free association, interpretation of the patient's symptoms and behaviour, and analysis of the transference.

Transference phenomena are the feelings, positive and negative, developed by the patient for the doctor. They have no realistic foundation in the present and are related to his feelings for significant figures, usually parental, in the past. Psychoanalysis, and indeed any kind of psychotherapy, makes use of these feelings, finding that intellectual interpretations of the patient's problems are insufficient and that emotional understanding, as relived in transference, is essential for improvement. As a practical procedure, psychoanalysis occupies some five daily hours each week over several years and is carried out by a psychoanalyst who himself has undertaken a lengthy and expensive training analysis. There are few analysts in the National Health Service and clearly they can treat only a handful of patients.

Psychoanalysis has been criticised as an unscientific theory but it has generated much clinical material and many ideas which have been proven or disproven by later research. Its influence in many fields other than psychiatry has been great. The efficacy of the technique is unproven. Freud had, and has many disciples some of whom, notably Alfred Adler (1870-1937) and Jung (1875-1961) broke with Freud to form their own schools. In modern psychotherapy there are many theoretical viewpoints but studies of psychotherapists show that whatever their theories their practices do not differ to any serious extent. Current practice leans toward more active participation by the therapist, concentration on the present rather than the past, and on analysis of transference and the patient's typical defence mechanisms rather than a search for traumatic events in the patient's childhood.

Indications for psychotherapy

Psychoneurosis and some personality and psychosomatic disorders. For intensive psychotherapy the patients selected are usually young, intelligent, highly-motivated, with an ability to verbalise freely and capacity for insight. Brief and supportive psychotherapy is used in all the milder psychiatric disorders.

Types of psychotherapy

Psychiatrists, and many others, practise psychotherapy of varying degrees of intensity, ranging from brief and infrequent interviews to weekly sessions of one hour continuing over months and years.

1. *Brief therapy*

A variety of techniques are exploited, usually in combination:

Ventilation, in which the patient confides, confesses, and is given the opportunity to ventilate his past and present difficulties.

Clarification, where problems are discussed and their nature and relations made clear.

Abreaction, verbalising emotionally charged material, with the release of anxiety, anger or grief.

Desensitisation, in which repetitive ventilation of feelings, as in mourning, has a therapeutic effect.

Suppression. The therapist acts in a directive and authoritarian way, using direct advice, orders, exhortation, persuasion and suggestion. Suggestibility may be increased by hypnosis or reinforced by drugs or placebos.

2. *Intensive psychotherapy*

Such treatment is usually practised by those with specialist training and includes psychoanalysis. In contrast to brief therapy the interviews are longer and more frequent. The therapist assumes a more neutral attitude, there is more detailed examination of the patient's past and present problems, and some analysis of the transference is used in the treatment.

3. *Group and family therapy*

Treating patients in small groups, usually of about eight people, is more economical than individual psychotherapy, and has advantages for patients with marked social and interpersonal difficulties. Similar mechanisms and transference reactions occur and are made use of by the therapist. Sessions are held weekly, last one to one-and-a-half hours, and continue for one to two years. Family therapy involves group sessions with all the members of a family attending, the treatment often shared by a male and female therapist.

4. *Administrative therapy*

Because interpersonal relationships are so important in the

genesis and treatment of psychiatric disorders, considerable attention is given nowadays to staff-patient relations in psychiatric hospitals and wards. The concept of the hospital as a *therapeutic community,* developed by Maxwell Jones, involved organising the hospital in a democratic way, with patients having a say in the conduct of their affairs, and staff relinquishing authoritarian habits. There must be free communications between doctors, nurses, other staff and patients, and all should feel able and have the opportunity to express their feelings to one another. To this end staff and patients meet regularly, and ward meetings become an extension of group psychotherapy. When such principles were neglected, patients became apathetic and experienced a loss of individuality, a condition which has been called *institutional neurosis.*

Behaviour therapy

Behaviour therapy has been developed from Pavlov's work on conditioning and from modern learning theories. In contrast to psychoanalytic theory psychoneurotic symptoms are regarded as learned responses which can be 'unlearned' by deconditioning the patient's responses.

The first technique used was *systematic desensitisation* in which the patient is trained to oppose feelings of anxiety by relaxing and then to face anxiety-producing situations (in reality or imagination) in graduated stages. Intravenous barbiturates may be used to aid relaxation. The results are good in single phobias (insects, flying) but less good in agoraphobia.

Aversion therapy uses mild electric shocks as a conditioning technique in alcoholism and sexual deviations. *Flooding (implosion therapy)* involves continuously exposing the patient in imagination or reality to feared situations or objects. *Operant conditioning* uses immediate rewards when the desired behaviour appears. Speech and actions can be 'shaped' and the technique is used in *token economies* where tokens, exchangeable for goods and privileges, are used as rewards in rehabilitating chronic patients. The effectiveness of all these techniques is the subject of much current research.

FURTHER READING

Psychotherapy cannot be learned entirely from books but even the student who has no wish to become a skilled therapist will improve his interviewing technique if he reads at least some of the following paperbacks:

Berne, E. *Games People Play*. Penguin.

Brown, J. A. C. *Freud and the Post Freudians*. Penguin.

Foulkes, S. H. & Anthony, E. J. *Group Psychotherapy*. Penguin.

Freud, S. *Two Short Accounts of Psychoanalysis*. Penguin.

Harris, T. A. *I'm OK — You're OK*. Pan.

Jones, E. (Ed. Trilling, L.) *Life and Work of Sigmund Freud*. Penguin.

Marcuse, F. L. *Hypnosis*. Penguin.

Meyer, V. & Chesser, E. S. *Behaviour Therapy in Clinical Psychiatry*. Penguin.

Stafford-Clark, D. *What Freud Really Said*. Penguin.

Walton, H. *Small Group Psychotherapy*. Penguin.

22. Physical Treatments

Physical treatments have developed rapidly in the last 40 years. Many are crude and empirical; some, like malarial therapy for cerebral syphilis and insulin coma therapy for schizophrenia have almost vanished; others, like ECT (electro-convulsive therapy) and psychosurgery have been refined and have survived. In the last 20 years the development of many new drugs has produced the specialty of psychopharmacology.

Psychopharmacology

The development and assessment of new drugs in psychiatry poses exceptional problems. Animal responses can provide only a rough comparison with possible effects on psychiatric symptoms, but many useful techniques exist. Motor behaviour, learning and memory, appetite and sexual activity can all be measured. Aggression in animals resembles irritability in man, and experimental neurosis (Pavlov) simulates fear and anxiety. As in some humans, the administration of reserpine to animals produces a state resembling retarded depression, which has been widely used to test the effects of new anti-depressants. The known effects of established psychotropic drugs on animals are utilised in screening new drugs.

In man, objective measures and rating scales are used when testing new drugs. Difficulties arise from the fluctuating course of many illnesses, and from lack of diagnostic precision, e.g. is a new drug for schizophrenia effective for all symptoms, in acute and chronic, hebephrenic and paranoid forms, etc.? The most serious obstacle of all is the *placebo reaction* arising from a number of non-specific factors, which may influence the patient's response:

  a. *Patient factors:* sex, age, symptoms, personality
  b. *Doctor factors:* the doctor's enthusiasm or lack of it has been shown to affect trial results

c. *Environment:* hospital or home, presence of other patients on the same drug

d. *Drug factors:* colour, taste, preparation (tablet, liquid, etc), frequency, route — injections have more impact than oral medication.

Some degree of placebo response can be found in two-thirds of patients (and healthy people) and is not confined to patients with neurosis or personality disorders.

No new drug becomes established today without adequate controlled trial ('double-blind') against a placebo or the established remedy. Side effects, toxic effects and the risk of dependency must also be measured.

1. Drug treatments

Tranquillisers

a. *Phenothiazine derivatives* are divided into three main groups according to side chain on phenothiazine nucleus:

(i) dimethylaminopropyl side chain
(ii) piperazine side chain
(iii) piperidine side chain.

Examples:

Group (i)	Chlorpromazine hydrochloride
Trade name:	Largactil.
Indications:	Controls agitation and excitement and is used in the treatment of schizophrenia, agitated depression, manic states, drug and alcohol withdrawal and delirium.
Dosage:	75-1000 mg daily. Available as tablets of 10, 25, 50 and 100 mg. Also 25 mg/ml solution for injection. Average dose 300 mg daily.
Side effects:	Tachycardia, postural hypotension, dry mouth, constipation, drowsiness, skin rashes and increased sensitivity to sunlight. Parkinsonism with large doses.
Toxic effects:	Impairment of liver function in 5-10 per cent of patients and more with high doses. Cholestatic jaundice in about 1 per cent. Agranulocytosis occurs rarely.
Group (ii)	Trifluoperazine
Trade name:	Stelazine.
Indications:	As for chlorpromazine. More potent but less sedative effect. Available as 1 mg and 5 mg tablets, and 2, 10 and 15 mg 'spansules'. Average dose in schizophrenia 5 mg thrice daily.

Side effects:	In doses over 15 mg daily extrapyramidal symptoms are common: Parkinsonism, dyskinesias, muscle spasm. Initial restless phase common.

Fluphenazine

Trade names:	Moditen, Modecate.
Indications:	As for chlorpromazine. Slow release preparations fluphenazine enanthate (Moditen Enanthate) and fluphenazine decanoate (Modecate) 25 mg per ml given every 2-4 weeks are now widely used for maintenance treatment of schizophrenics — especially on an out-patient or day-patient basis.
Side effects:	Extra-pyramidal symptoms are common with the slow release forms and an anti-Parkinson drug (e.g. orphenadrine (Disipal) 150-300 mg daily) may be needed in addition.

Group (iii)   Thioridazine hydrochloride

Trade name:	Melleril.
Indications:	As for chlorpromazine.
Dosage:	Up to 600 mg daily.
Side effects:	May be less frequent than with other phenothiazines.

Many other phenothiazine derivatives are on the market. These have no marked advantage over the examples mentioned above.

Group (i)   Promazine (Sparine)
           Methotrimeprazine (Veractil)
   (ii) Prochlorperazine (Stemetil)
           Perphenazine (Fentazin)
  (iii) Pericyazine (Neulactil).

b. *Benzodiazepine group*

Examples:
Chlordiazepoxide

Trade name:	Librium.
Indications:	Anxiety and tension. Probably compares well with barbiturates. Said to be useful in obsessional and phobic states.
Dosage:	10-20 mg t.i.d.
Side effects:	Dizziness, nausea, disinhibited behaviour seen occasionally.

Other members of this group include:
Oxazepam (Serenid) 10-30 mg t.i.d.
Diazepam (Valium) 2-10 mg t.i.d.
Medazepam (Nobrium) 5-10 mg t.i.d.
Nitrazepam (Mogadon) 5-10 mg at night.
Lorazepam (Ativan) 1-2.5 mg t.i.d.
Flurazepam (Dalmane) 15-30 mg at night.

c. *Miscellaneous group.* Many other tranquillising drugs are available and widely used. It is preferable to become

familiar with the side effects and dosage of a few than to change too frequently.

Some popular members of the group are:

Chlormethiazole (Heminevrin) 0.5-1.0 g t.i.d. Often used for delirium and in the elderly. Some risk of dependence.

Haloperidol (Serenace) 0.5-5 mg t.i.d. Useful in acute mania.

Flupenthixol (Depixol) 20-40 mg i.m. every 2 to 4 weeks. Used in chronic schizophrenia.

Pimozide (Orap) 2-10 mg daily. Used in schizophrenia. Advantage of single daily dose.

Fluspiriline (Redeptin) 2-8 mg i.m. every 1 to 2 weeks in schizophrenia.

Antidepressant compounds
a. Imino-dibenzyl group
Imipramine hydrochloride

Trade names:	Tofranil, Berkomine.
Pharmacology:	An imino-dibenzyl derivative. It has both anti-cholinergic and adrenergic effects. It has no euphoriant effect when given to normal subjects. Its exact mode of action is unknown but it raises the levels of serotonin and catecholamines in the brain and produces EEG changes in the diencephalon where these substances are in their highest concentration. Other experimental evidence suggests that catecholamines play an important role in mood regulation.
Indications:	Imipramine can in most cases replace ECT. It is effective in endogenous depression, but less often helps reactive depressions. Retarded patients respond better than those who are agitated. Patients respond gradually in from one to four weeks, which is a disadvantage in potentially suicidal cases. Over 50 per cent of the endogenous depressions remit but relapse occurs if a maintenance dose is not given.
Dosage:	25-75 mg t.i.d.
Side effects:	Dry mouth and difficulty in focusing (anti-cholinergic), attacks of sweating and flushing (adrenergic) are all common. Less commonly and with doses over 200 mg daily, tremors, muscle twitchings, dysuria and epilepsy (1-2 per cent). Headaches, insomnia and slight hypotension may occur. Some patients may become hypomanic during treatment. Cardiotoxic effects also found.

Amitriptyline hydrochloride

Trade names:	Tryptizol, Saroten, Laroxyl, Lentizol ('spansule').
Pharmacology:	Similar to imipramine but has some phenothiazine-like action.
Indications:	As for imipramine, useful for agitated depression.
Dosage:	25-75 mg t.i.d. 25-100 mg spansules at night.
Side effects:	As for imipramine.

Others

Opipramol (Insidon), trimipramine (Surmontil), desipramine (Pertofan), nortriptyline (Aventyl, Allegron), dibenzepin (Noveril), doxepin (Sinequan), iprindole (Prondol), clomipramine (Anafranil), protriptyline (Concordin).

b. *Amine-oxidase inhibitors*

Phenelzine

Trade name:	Nardil
Pharmacology:	A hydrazine derivative. The action in depression is probably due to the ability to inhibit amine-oxidase. The function of the enzyme monoamine-oxidase is the breakdown of serotonin and catecholamines in the brain. Amine-oxidase inhibitors consequently raise the brain levels of serotonin and catecholamines.
Indications:	Atypical or milder depressions, especially with evening worsening and phobias.
Dosage:	15-30 mg t.i.d.
Side effects:	Dizziness, hypotension, hepatitis, urinary retention. Severe headache with hypertension may occur, often after eating cheese and other substances rich in tyramine due to the inhibition of amine-oxidase and the pressor effects of the tyramine.
Precautions:	Patients on this group drugs must avoid cheese, meat extracts, peas and beans, alcohol, ephedrine, pethidine. Because of these precautions the drug should not be used unless no other form of treatment is appropriate.

Others

Isocarboxazid (Marplan), tranylcypromine (Parnate), nialamide (Niamid). There is no convincing evidence that any one of these is more effective than any other amine-oxidase inhibitor.

c. *Tryptophan*

L-tryptophan (Optimax) 2-6 g/day is used in some cases of depression. Results are still being assessed.

d. *Lithium*

Lithium carbonate (Camcolit) or in a delayed release tablet (Priadel) is effective in treating mania and is used increasingly to prevent relapse in manic-depressive psychosis. Because of the toxicity — (drowsiness, ataxia, vomiting) — renal and thyroid function must be checked before starting treatment and serum levels must be monitored (to 0.6-1.2 meq./l). The average patient requires about 1200 mg daily. In patients with an established history of manic depressive psychosis or recurrent depression and who can be relied upon to co-operate, this drug given indefinitely will significantly reduce the risk of relapse or readmission to hospital. However, reports of toxicity are frequent and the drug administration should be supervised at an appropriate clinic.

Hypnotics and sedatives

These drugs are administered for the symptomatic relief of insomnia, agitation and panic.

a. Benzodiazepines (see p. 111)

Nitrazepam (Mogadon) 5-10 mg is a safe and reliable hypnotic for the treatment of insomnia.

b. Barbiturates

Duration of action depends on stability of side-chain, tissue absorption and rate of kidney excretion. They are detoxicated in the liver.

Dangers: Addiction; suicidal attempts; skin sensitivity reactions. Barbiturates are best avoided in psychiatry where the duration of illness increases risk of habituation.

c. Chloralhydrate

Inexpensive and relatively safe. Gastric irritation is an occasional drawback. *Dose:* 1-2 g.

Other suitable preparations include dichloralphenazone (Welldorm) as tablet or elixir (1-2, 650 mg tabs, 10-20 ml elixir) and triclofos (Tricloryl) as tablet or syrup (1-2 g, 10-20 ml).

d. Promethazine hydrochloride (Phenergan)

An anti-histamine with an hypnotic side effect.
Dose: 25-50 mg tablets or elixir.

e. Paraldehyde

A safe but unpleasant hypnotic: malodorous breath.
Dose: 2-10 ml orally or intramuscularly. Now used only in status epilepticus, delirium or severe mania. Must be given by a glass syringe.

f. Doriden (Glutethimide)

Said to be safe and relatively non-addictive. May cause nausea and skin rash.
Dose: 0.25-0.5 g.

g. Morphine/Hyoscine

Valuable for acutely restless or violent case.
Dose: Morphine sulphate 15 mg with hyoscine hydrobromide 0.6 mg.

2. Electro-convulsive therapy (ECT)

Can be given to suitable patients in out-patient departments as well as in hospital. Given bilaterally or unilaterally.

Method

1. Physical examination with special reference to chest and heart disease.

2. Proper psychological preparation, giving patient clear indication of what will happen. Privacy during treatment and presence of familiar figures on recovery are helpful.

3. Patient's/relative's consent for treatment.

4. 'Anaesthetic' breakfast: empty bowel and bladder: remove dentures.

5. Atropine sulphate, 0.6 mg 45-60 minutes before treatment.

6. To modify convulsion give intravenous thiopentone (Pentothal: 0.25-0.5 g) followed by suxamethonium chloride (Scoline: about 50 mg) under supervision of anaesthetist. Insufflation of oxygen necessary until respiration is restored.

7. Induce convulsion by introduction of electric current via saline pad electrodes across temples. (The stimulus is of the order of 140 volts for 0.5 seconds.) This is 'bilateral' ECT.

Duration of treatment

Usually two per week; total number gauged by patient's response; four to ten in depressed patients.

Contraindications

Serious cardiovascular disease, peptic ulcer, pulmonary tuberculosis. These contraindications are not absolute and must be weighed against likely benefit.

Indications

1. Endogenous depression (manic-depressive depression).

2. Mania — occasionally successful in very acute cases. Much less successful in hypomania.

3. Acute schizophrenia where affective disturbance prominent — usually in association with phenothiazine drugs.

4. Certain cases of intractable hypochondriasis.

5. Rarely, to terminate delirious states or epileptic psychoses.

3. Insulin

Modified insulin or insulin subcoma treatment

Slight or moderate state of hypoglycaemia is induced. Give soluble insulin, 10-50 units, at 7 a.m. (not enough to produce coma) and feed at 9.30 or 10 a.m. Often valuable in severe chronic anxiety neurosis, reactive depression with recent weight loss and in anorexia nervosa.

4. Psychosurgery

History

In the late 1940's thousands of patients were treated by standard leucotomy — a blind procedure by which the frontal white matter was divided with a blunt instrument through temporal burr-holes. The operation relieved anxiety, depressive and obsessional symptoms but often led to crippling after-effects, notably epilepsy and serious personality change, with severe apathy or disinhibition. It was virtually abandoned during the 1950's. In the last 25 years many modified procedures have been developed.

Anatomy

Emotional experience has been shown to be closely linked to the *limbic system,* comprising the hippocampus, amygdalum, fornix, the hippocampal and cingulate gyri, and the posterior part of the orbital frontal cortex. This system has complex connections with the frontal lobes, the hypothalamus and the brain stem. Current psychosurgery aims to produce limited lesions in the limbic system or its connections.

Techniques

a. Undercutting of the medial third of the orbital cortex

b. Bimedial leucotomy — aimed at the fronto-thalamic bundle

c. Cingulectomy — anterior cingulate gyrus

d. Stereotactic lesions. Many are being tested, e.g. lesions in the subcaudate nucleus, amygdala, thalamus and hypothalamus. All the above operations are bilateral.

Risks

Operative mortality is now negligible, and because of the limited lesions produced and stringent selection of patients, epilepsy and undesirable personality change are rare.

Indications

a. Symptoms are a better guide than diagnosis. Tension, severe anxiety, chronic depression and obsessional symptoms respond best to surgery

b. Operation is not carried out until other treatments have failed, but should not be unduly delayed

c. Older patients improve more than the young

d. In temporal lobe epilepsy (see p. 35) associated behavioural disturbance may be improved by surgery.

Results

In patients selected carefully the operations are successful in the majority of cases. At best there is complete symptomatic relief; even if this is not achieved the patient is able to benefit from rehabilitation and may respond to other treatments which had previously failed.

FURTHER READING

Claridge, G. S. *Drugs and Human Behaviour*. Penguin.

23. Psychiatric Emergencies

Uncommon in general practice, frequent in casualty departments, psychiatric emergencies are worrying and time-consuming when they occur. In handling them a few general principles are crucial:

1. *Attitude.* However disturbed the behaviour of the patient, or those about him, behave calmly and quietly and seem confident and unhurried.

2. *Honesty.* Never lie to the patient or agree to any subterfuge relatives may suggest, e.g. pretending not to be a doctor, or that the patient is not being sent to a psychiatric hospital.

3. *History-taking.* The more disturbed the patient, the more helpful it is to take a short history from a relative or neighbour before seeing him.

4. *Use of force — compulsory admission.* Before using or advising physical restraint, the doctor should examine the patient, preferably alone. Most disturbed patients settle in a quiet atmosphere with a competent interviewer, but in the few cases where the patient's behaviour remains violent, unco-operative and an obvious danger to himself and others, there should be no delay in giving needed treatment, usually sedation prior to compulsory admission to hospital. If restraint is needed, a more than adequate number of assistants should be used, to reduce the risk of injury on both sides. Half measures are worse than useless.

Some common emergencies

Acute stress reactions

Panic, weeping, 'hysterics' and other signs of distress are often seen after personal or social disasters such as bereavements and bombings. They are quickly relieved by a period of sleep achieved by adequate doses of hypnotics, e.g.

amylobarbitone sod. 200 to 400 mg orally. Such psychiatric casualties must be envisaged in all major disaster plans. Adequate treatment diminishes subsequent post-traumatic neurosis, and if not available interferes with the treatment of other victims.

Acute agitation

Agitation may be seen in phobic and anxiety states and in depressive illness. Severe neurotic emergencies are best managed by a single large oral or parenteral dose of a barbiturate, or a benzodiazepine. In agitated depression, chlorpromazine, 50 mg intramuscularly is often effective.

Paranoid delusions

Delusions of persecution may be the presenting symptom in schizophrenia, depression or senile psychoses. The patient may lock himself in his house to protect himself against his persecutors and entry may have to be forced with the help of relatives or the police. The patient may then agree to come to hospital although he may not admit that he is ill. In these suspicious patients a blunt, frank and honest approach is usually rewarded.

Alcohol and drugs

The noisy drunk may require the presence of the police for co-operation. An emetic may be used to hasten sobriety: drugs should be avoided. Always remember that drunkenness may conceal physical and psychiatric illness; head injury, depression and parasuicide are examples.

Drug abuse may present with the 'bad trip' of the L.S.D. taker, the drunken gait and speech of the barbiturate taker, or the flushed hyperactivity of the amphetamine abuser. Phenothiazines should be given for L.S.D. reactions, and appropriate treatment for the others as necessary.

The drug addict taking heroin, opiates, etc. is usually young, aggressive, demanding, untruthful and persistent in his demands for supplies. He is usually knowledgeable about his condition and legal rights. If he claims to be a registered addict this should be checked with the Home Office who keep registers and provide a telephone service. Only methadone should be given, in a single dose of 5 to 10 mg seen to be taken, and the patient should then be referred to the nearest official clinic for addicts.

Suicidal attempts

Medical or surgical treatment of the emergency obviously takes precedence, but information about the circumstances should be collected at the time — it may be concealed or difficult to obtain later. On recovery the depressed patient often feels better temporarily, or may conceal his persistent suicidal thoughts. All parasuicides should have a psychiatric examination.

The violent and hostile patient

Such situations are extremely rare but may occur in acute mania, catatonic excitement, paranoid schizophrenia, some acute organic states, and in epileptic furor. Restraint, sedation and compulsory admission will usually be needed. The best emergency sedative in such cases is an injection of chlorpromazine 50 to 100 mg given through the clothing if need be. Morphine may be substituted if chlorpromazine is not available. In organic confusion, especially in epilepsy and in the elderly, paraldehyde 5 to 10 ml intramuscularly is effective and safe but smelly. For the noisy drunk apomorphine 5 to 8 mg is effective.

Hypomanic patients who are insightless and overcheerful may be irritable and hostile for short periods, especially when admission is suggested. Given time and patience they can usually be coaxed into co-operation. This is rarely feasible in acute schizophrenic and organic states, where if treatment is urgently indicated there should be no hesitation in ensuring that it is obtained, if necessary by compulsory admission.

24. Rehabilitation

Much mental illness is chronic and seriously affects the patient's social and occupational performance. Psychiatric hospitals usually house large numbers of patients suffering from chronic schizophrenia and for these and other patients programmes of social and occupational rehabilitation are essential. For the rehabilitation of psychiatric patients the creation of a *'treatment team'* is necessary. Psychiatrist, nurse, social worker, psychologist, occupational therapist and, to a smaller extent, physiotherapist and speech therapist will all have a part to play. Many psychiatric hospitals have developed the idea of a *'therapeutic community'* in which all members of staff and patients meet regularly to discuss day-to-day problems and to help patients with their social difficulties. Programmes of work for patients help to restore confidence and to create a more realistic pattern of daily living. Most psychiatric hospitals now have *industrial therapy* departments where patients work regular hours for some financial reward. Patients whose work performance improves will often be referred to an *industrial rehabilitation unit* (run by the Department of Employment and Productivity) where the patient's working capacity is assessed and his ability to return to normal employment can be demonstrated. In addition to social and occupational programmes most mental health services now have a proportion of day patients. Patients suffering from chronic mental illness are encouraged to leave hospital and to return by day. Patients normally return to their own homes but where there is no suitable home, lodgings or a hostel provided by the local authority are used. The administration of long-acting phenothiazine drugs (see p. 111) to chronic schizophrenic patients has increased the number able to live outwith hospital.

The Mental Health Acts gave local authorities statutory responsibility to provide services for the mentally ill living in the community. Most local authorities provided some social work and nursing services but few provided residential or day care. The Social Work Acts extend this responsibility for community mental health services and there has been some increased provision of community services for the mentally ill by social work departments. However, such developments have been slow and the psychiatric services continue to provide the major part of the mental health service. The contribution of social work to rehabilitation is of considerable importance. The social worker is trained to assess the social and family problems of the patient and to give advice about the services available to help. Social workers are also trained to help with the emotional problems of patients and their families and there should be constant co-operation between the social worker and the doctor.

Further reading

The student of psychiatry is well served by a large number of paperbacks on special subjects. Most of the books suggested at the end of chapters are in this form and relatively cheap. A selection should be made according to the student's interests or on the recommendation of teachers. Those in controversial fields, in areas where there are recent advances and on psychotherapy are particularly valuable.

Many short general textbooks are available. We recommend:

Merskey, H. & Tonge, W. L. *Psychiatric Illness,* Bailliere, Tindall & Cox which deals capably with minor psychiatry and the elements of psychotherapy.

Hays, P. *New Horizons in Psychiatry,* Penguin, is a painless introduction to contemporary psychiatry.

In clinical work and for reference the student should refer to larger texts or find his way to original papers. He should consult:

Slater & Roth. *Clinical Psychiatry.* Cassell, which is the standard British textbook and:

Sim, M. *Guide to Psychiatry.* Churchill Livingstone which is lively and has extensive references.

Granville-Grossman, K. *Recent Advances in Clinical Psychiatry.* Churchill.

Tredgold, R. F. & Soddy, K. *Textbook of Mental Deficiency.* Bailliere, Tindall & Cox.

Glossary

Some of the terms used in these notes may be unfamiliar to students or used in an unfamiliar sense. The following explanations indicate how the terms are used in the notes and are not strict definitions. Definitions of other technical words and phrases can be traced by using the index.

Abstract thinking. The ability to use concepts and ideas independently of concrete objects.

Acalculia. Loss of the ability to calculate.

Affect. Mood, feeling or emotion.

Agraphia. Loss of the ability to write.

Alexia. Loss of the ability to read.

Anterograde amnesia. Inability to remember events occurring *after* a brain injury, even though the patient was apparently conscious (cf. retrograde amnesia).

Aphasia (dysphasia). Loss or partial loss of the ability to use language (i.e. to speak or to recognise the spoken word).

Asthenic build. Tall slender body-shape (cf. pyknic).

Autistic thinking. Thinking which is unduly self-directed.

Confabulation. False recall associated with failure in memory.

Constitution. The total hereditary characteristics of a person.

Conversion. The mechanism whereby anxiety is transformed into a physical symptom.

Compulsion. An impulse to carry out or repeat certain actions resisted by the patient and usually recognised by him as meaningless.

Curator Bonis. A person appointed by the Courts in Scotland to look after a patient's affairs when he is incapable of doing so himself or of directing others to do so.

Delirium. Transitory or potentially reversible mental confusion.

Delusions. False beliefs or attitudes with no basis in reality, often illogical.

Dementia. The end-stage of intellectual deterioration. An irreversible state of brain damage.

Depersonalisation. A feeling that one has lost one's feelings or identity or that one is unreal.

Derealisation. A feeling that things in the environment are no longer real.

Dereistic thinking. Thinking concerned with phantastic or imaginary events.

Dissociation. A process whereby certain psychological activities lose their relationship to the remainder of the personality and function more or less independently.

Dysarthria. Faulty articulation of speech.

Dysmnesia. Partial disturbance of memory (cf. amnesia).

Echopraxia. Automatic and purposeless imitation of another person's movements.

Euphoria. Mood of well-being, sometimes inappropriate (e.g. in presence of physical illness).

Extraversion. The general characteristic of those individuals whose interests and reactions are directed outwards (cf. introversion where interests are predominantly directed inwards).

Fetishism. Condition in which sexual excitement is aroused by the presence of a non-sexual object.

Hallucination. Convincing perception in any sensory modality (e.g. vision, hearing, taste, smell, touch) independent of the relevant stimulation (cf. illusion).

Hypochondriasis. Morbid concern with health or with bodily processes.

Illusion. Mistaken perception in any sensory modality (cf. hallucination).

Incidence. The number of cases of an illness which arise in a population in a given period (cf. prevalence).

Integration of personality. The extent to which an individual's personal qualities are unified or consistent.

Knight's move thinking. Reasoning which omits an essential step.

Libido. Sexual drive or urge.

Neologism. A specially coined or nonsensical word (e.g. 'brillig').

Neurasthenia. Term applied to neurotic disorder characterised by weakness and fatiguability.

Neuroticism. The tendency or predisposition of an individual to become neurotic.

Obsession. A dominating and repetitive experience or idea which cannot be resisted even although recognised as senseless.

Oedipal situation. Freud's explanation, based on the story of King Oedipus, of the emotional indentifications within the family. The son identified with father has strong emotional ties with mother.

Orientation. Knowledge of one's identity and one's situation in place and time and in regard to other persons.

Paranoid. Literally, false reasoning. Having delusions, usually of persecution. *Paranoid personality* — an individual who is suspicious and sensitive.

Perseveration. Persistence or recurrence of an idea or action. Inability to shift from one task to another.

Personality. All the unique personal qualities of an individual.

Phantasticant. Drug which produces phantastic experiences, such as visual hallucinations, in normal individuals.

Prevalence. The amount of an illness which exists in a population at a particular time (cf. incidence).

Psychiatric social worker. A specially trained social worker who is responsible for investigating and remedying the patient's social, family and occupational circumstances.

Psychodynamics. The study of the way in which past experiences and attitudes produce present symptoms.

Psychopathology. The study of the ideas and experiences which occur in psychological disorders.

Pyknic build. Short thick-set body shape (cf. asthenic).

Rapport. Mutually confident relationship between two people (e.g. patient and doctor).

Retrograde amnesia. Inability to remember events occurring *prior to* a brain injury or to brain damage due to an acute illness (cf. anterograde amnesia).

Sado-masochism. Sexual gratification aroused by inflicting pain (sadism) or suffering pain (masochism).

Siblings. Children of the same parents.

Stereotyped act. A uniform, persistent and repetitive sequence of behaviour, usually having no purpose.

Transvestism. Condition in which sexual gratification is obtained from wearing clothing of the opposite sex.

Volition. The act of deciding upon and initiating a course of action.

Index